# Planning and Positioning in MRI

For my parents, Jack and Irene, who gave each of their children the only real inheritance that matters—
a sound education and an open and tolerant mind.

# Planning and Positioning in MRI

## Anne Bright

Grad Dip MRI, BAppSc
MRI Supervisor, North Shore Radiology & Nuclear Medicine
Member Australian Institute of Radiography (AIR)
Member of Section for Magnetic Resonance Technologists (SMRT)

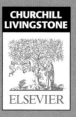

CHURCHILL
LIVINGSTONE

ELSEVIER

Sydney     Edinburgh     London     New York     Philadelphia     St Louis     Toronto

Churchill Livingstone
is an imprint of Elsevier

Elsevier Australia. ACN 001 002 357
(a division of Reed International Books Australia Pty Ltd)
Tower 1, 475 Victoria Avenue, Chatswood, NSW 2067

National Library of Australia Cataloguing-in-Publication Data

---

Bright, Anne.

Planning and positioning in MRI / Anne Bright.

1st ed.

9780729539852 (pbk.)
    Includes index.
    Magnetic resonance imaging.
    Magnetic resonance imaging—Diagnostic use.

616.07548

---

Publisher: Melinda McEvoy
Developmental Editor: Rebecca Cornell
Publishing Services Manager: Helena Klijn
Project Coordinator: Natalie Hamad
Edited by Brenda Hamilton
Proofread by Sarah Newton-John
Cover and internal design by Lewis Tsalis
Index by Robert Swanson
Typeset by Toppan Best-set Premedia Limited
Printed by China Translation & Printing Services Ltd.

# Contents

| Section 1 | Head and neck |
|-----------|---------------|

| Section 2 | Spine |
|-----------|-------|

| Section 3 | Chest and abdomen |
|-----------|-------------------|

# Introduction

When commencing in magnetic resonance imaging, the range of pulse sequences, variable appearances of pathology and image orientation may overwhelm trainees. The approach taken in the writing of this text reflects the intended audience, namely radiographers actually performing the examination, operating the scanner. Most, if not all sites are under the direction of a radiologist who prescribes pulse sequences and ultimately reports on the outcomes, but it is the radiographer sitting at the operator console who must know the imaging planes and degree of coverage required, just as they would for an X-ray or CT examination. This text aims to address this issue, focusing upon patient positioning and image planning, with a limited description of what may be demonstrated in each scan plane.

MRI is dictated not only by anatomical region, but also by pathological extent and body habitus. While each site will have a preferred approach for scanning each body region, there are basic principles that can be learned. Once the basic principles of good positioning are developed, what was once purely rote knowledge will become applied wisdom, establishing the foundations necessary for the lateral thought processes necessary to manage complex cases.

A detailed discussion of physics, scan parameters and safety is outside the scope of this text. Most sites will have routine scans programmed for their most common examinations. Nevertheless, a brief overview of some of the considerations required in building a pulse sequence follows and should be borne in mind by the trainee. More detailed information is available in the many excellent resources already available both in print and via the internet.

Kinematic imaging of the joints is beyond the scope of this text, but is a useful adjunct in the examination of joint instabilities and impingements. Generally, a non-ferromagnetic device is required to fix the proximal portion of the joint, while allowing a radiographer to alter the position of the distal joint incrementally.

The text endeavours to include images that demonstrate slice orientation on anatomy that is not distorted by disease. In cases where pathology may be evident, image selection has been made to assist the student in learning the principles that underpin good positioning and anatomical coverage. The majority of scanners are superconducting, requiring a patient to lie on a table, and the text is written from such a perspective. Nevertheless, the guidelines concerning anatomical coverage and demonstrated structures do not change, being pertinent regardless of scanner design.

A final note on terms. Debate exists over the appropriate term for the person operating the MRI scanner. This is partially due to variations in terms between the various jurisdictions and the relative qualifications. It includes terms such as radiographer, operator, imaging practitioner, technician and technologist. The term radiographer is used throughout this text as an all-encompassing means of inclusion for all individuals performing MRI scans, regardless of their affiliation.

## Safety

The importance of vigilance in screening every person who enters the MRI environment cannot be overstated. Careful and repeated screening (at the time of booking, when registering at reception, when changing and before entering the scan room) by the staff at each point provides the best opportunity to prevent injury to the patient, support companions and staff.

Not all sites ask a patient to change into a cotton or disposable paper examination gown, although this is to be encouraged. This simple requirement dramatically reduces the possibility of a patient entering the scan room with objects in their pockets that may be rendered obsolete by the high field strength (e.g. credit cards) or may pose a threat as a projectile (e.g. keys, pocket knife). In combination with removing dental implants and all jewellery, a patient divested of all metal ensures maximal field homogeneity to achieve best image quality, as well as limiting the possibility of thermal injury due to items heating during scanning. Even the most benign-appearing metallic thread (e.g. lurex) can limit image quality or result in burns. Heavy make-up, especially around the eye, should also be removed, particularly when imaging the head to prevent image distortion. It's worth keeping a bottle of make-up remover in your unit. Caution with permanent make-up or tattoos, especially around the eyes, is necessary. These common preparation concepts, while not repeated throughout this text, should be borne in mind when preparing a patient and the examination room.

Padding is used to prevent conductive loops forming between skin surfaces, such as at the thighs or ankles. Wherever two skin surfaces meet or the skin touches the bore, there is potentially a conductive loop; place a MRI sponge between the two surfaces.

Hands on the body or above the head should be separated, and thermal padding placed between the patient and the bore of the magnet to prevent contact and possible thermal injury. Note that not all padding is MR-safe and some may pose a threat under certain circumstances. Only sponges supplied by a reputable MR supplier should be used within the scan room.

Hearing protection should be provided when operating a scanner that produces significant noise. Earplugs and/or muffs may be supplemented by padding around the head to further minimise noise. This will also aid in preventing patient motion during scans of the head or neck.

Supporting relatives or companions should be screened carefully to ensure that they have removed all potentially hazardous items and are wearing only simple clothing; no belts, no jewellery, nothing in the hair, pockets emptied.

Considerations for patient safety include checking the renal function of patients who will be administered gadolinium-based contrast media, especially when indications point toward renal disease. There is a burgeoning volume of information related to both contrast media and implant safety. The reader is directed to the many excellent resources available, often at very little cost. A list of suggested support resources may be found at the end of this introduction.

## Artefacts

As with any radiological examination, motion will degrade image quality. Making the patient as comfortable as possible will minimise the potential for motion. Supporting limbs, padding around the head, placing a sponge under the knees to alleviate back pain, can all assist in preventing patient motion. Again, use only padding supplied by a reputable MRI vendor. Do not grab a sandbag from the nearest X-ray room—it's not always just sand!

Another common artefact encountered by the trainee in MRI is phase wrap (aliasing). Always check the phase direction and assess whether the field of view is sufficient to encompass the anatomy. If not, there are three options—changing the phase direction, increasing the field of view or applying phase oversampling (no phase wrap). Each of these carries a potential cost; be sure you are aware of the impact of making a change.

Ghosting is due to the pulsation of arterial flow causing tracks across an image in the phase direction. Again, altering the phase direction so that the artefact does not track over the anatomy of interest may be an acceptable remedy, but perhaps better would be applying a saturation pulse just outside the field of view to null the signal of inflowing blood. In the head and neck, the saturation pulse would be placed inferiorly to null blood as it flows into the head; in the rest of the body, the pulse would generally be applied superior to the field of view.

A saturation pulse is also helpful in nulling the signal from respiratory motion in the abdomen. Images of the abdomen and pelvis will often benefit from a saturation pulse applied over the subcutaneous fat of the abdomen or diaphragm. For imaging of the spine, a saturation pulse placed just anterior to the vertebra will reduce artefact from swallowing and aortic pulsation, but be careful not to saturate the signal if there is a paraspinal lesion.

There are many other artefacts that may be encountered, including but not limited to truncation, Gibb's artefact and chemical shift. These are less related to patient position and slice orientation. A comprehensive description, explanation and management strategy for each of these and many other MRI artefacts can be found in a physics text.

# Image weighting

Image weighting is a function of pulse repetition time (TR) and echo time (TE) (see table below), combined with the method employed to generate the echo. Rapid acquisition and relaxation enhancement (RARE, also known as fast spine echo, turbo spin echo) produces true T2 image contrast, the refocusing pulses minimising the effects of field inhomogeneities. Gradient echo (GRE, also known as fast field echo) using refocusing gradient pulses does not compensate for the effects of field inhomogeneities, generating T2* contrast. In addition, RARE employs a 90° excitation pulse (or nearly 90°), while GRE uses a much lower flip angle, anywhere between 10° and 60°. These fundamental differences impact on scan time, image quality and most importantly, image characteristics.

It is the combination of signal characteristics demonstrated on images in multiple imaging planes that assists in the determination of disease aetiology and differential diagnosis. While inhomogeneities generated by metallic implants such as spinal fusion or dental implants will degrade image quality, distorting anatomy and ruining fat saturation, this feature can be exploited to better demonstrate pathological processes such as microscopic bleeds in the brain or iron loading in the liver.

The fundamental difference in pulse sequence designs results in entirely differing parameters. In addition, field strength impacts on parameter values. Regardless of whether there are pre-loaded scans on your scanner, there will be occasions where you will be required to 'build' or manipulate a pulse sequence to meet the requirements of the particular pathology you are examining, or to ameliorate artefactual signal anomalies. The radiographer must be familiar with the appropriate range of parameters for the field strength at which they operate and for the specific type of pulse being used.

# Imaging coils

Defining anatomical boundaries for MRI provides a means of determining the area for inclusion when choosing an appropriate radiofrequency coil and planning a pulse sequence. Each imaging coil will have a specified field of view that must be taken into account by the radiographer when selecting an appropriate device. Many coils are designed with a particular task in mind, but are generally adapted in clinical use for imaging of more than one region of the body.

| Image weighting | Repetition time (TR) | Echo time (TE) |
|---|---|---|
| T1 | Short | Short |
| Proton density (PD) | Long | Short |
| T2/T2* | Long | Long |

Radiofrequency coil design has developed dramatically, and this will no doubt continue. Many sites still use older designs producing images of high spatial and contrast resolution. The radiographer needs to be aware of which coils are receive-only and which are transmit–receive. A receive-only coil detects emitted radiofreqency from the body after excitation has been induced by the intrinsic body coil incorporated in the scanner itself. In contrast, a transmit–receive coil both generates the excitation radiofreqency pulse and receives the emitted signal.

Various coil designs exploiting the benefits of combining coil elements have been developed. Linear polarised, circular (quadrature) polarised and phased array coils all have their own advantages and limitations, which can be studied elsewhere. The important thing to remember is that the protons closest to the imaging coil generate the highest signal. Detecting signal from protons deep within the tissues (e.g. within the abdomen) requires a coil of larger dimensions, but this also increases noise. Hence, selecting a coil with a field of view and physical design that best fits the region of interest is the first step in maximising image signal. The imaging coils that follow are used as examples only of the various forms and designs available.

Coils such as those in Figures I.1 and I.2 are suitable for imaging when a large field of view is required.

While these coils are suitable for imaging of the body (e.g. chest, heart, abdomen, hamstrings), they may also be used when patient body habitus or illness places constraints on traditional positioning. For example, a patient who is unable to lie on their back for an examination of the thoracic spine, may better tolerate the procedure when allowed to lie decubitus and imaged using a coil such as that in Figure I.1.

Breast imaging is performed prone, the breasts hanging into a cavity surrounded by elements built into the coil (Fig. I.3). These coils may include stabilising paddles. Compression is not required for MRI of the breast; the paddles simply serve as a

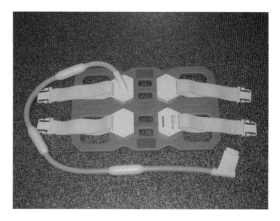

Figure I.2  Body matrix (Siemens).

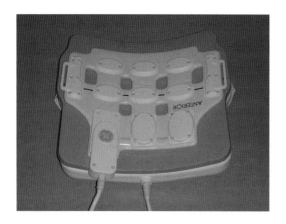

Figure I.1  8-channel cardiac array (GE Healthcare).

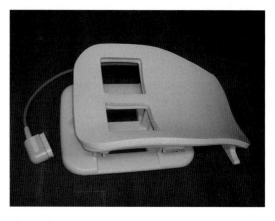

Figure I.3  SENSE breast coil 7 elements (Philips).

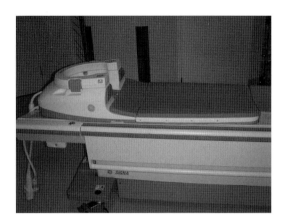

Figure I.4 16-channel head-neck-spine coil (GE Healthcare).

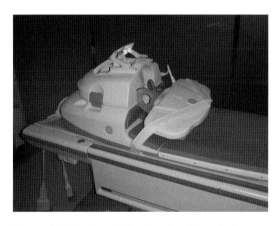

Figure I.5 16-channel head-neck-spine coil, face and chest elements (GE Healthcare).

means of preventing movement during image acquisition. Patients in whom a lesion is detected may require a MR biopsy, so perforated grids would be used in place of compression. These would typically be applied with more pressure.

Some coils have a modular design, allowing the radiographer to add elements to increase the field of view for imaging large regions of interest. Figure I.4 is set up to image the spine, but includes anterior elements (Fig I.5) for imaging of the head and brachial plexus. Figure I.6 shows two coils composing 16 coil elements in total; 12 coil elements for the

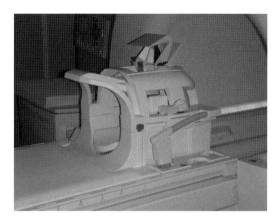

Figure I.6 Head and neck matrix coils (Siemens).

head and 4 coil elements for the neck parts respectively. The picture also shows the superior end of the spine coil attached to the head and neck coils. The neck coil may be removed if only an examination of the head is needed, although it many remain in place even if you don't need it for a particular exam. More coils with correspondingly more elements may be added to these two coils if greater coverage is needed.

The longer the examination duration, the more uncomfortable a patient may become. The ability to combine elements for multi-region imaging increases the utility of the individual coil modules, and makes imaging of multiple pathologies or clinical indications less cumbersome for the radiographer and decreases examination times.

Joints between long bones are best examined using coils designed for the region of interest. Imaging of the knee or elbow, using the 'Superman' position described in Chapter 5.2, may be performed with coils such as those in Figures I.7 and I.8. The chimney in the coil in Figure I.8 makes it suitable for also imaging the ankle and foot, although dedicated foot and ankle coils have also been designed (Fig I.9). A wrist coil is shown in Figure I.10.

A flexible coil (Fig I.11) is available in two sizes. It enables imaging of anatomy that may be distorted

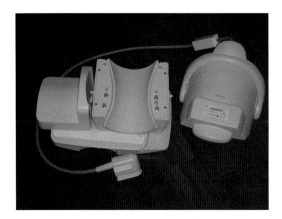

Figure I.7  SENSE knee coil 8 elements (Philips).

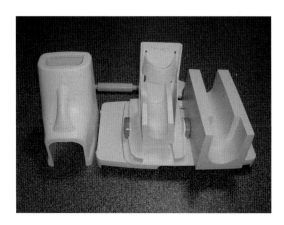

Figure I.9  InVivo 8-channel foot and ankle coil (Siemens).

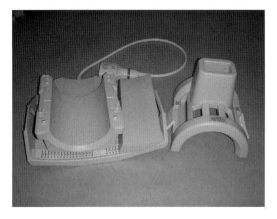

Figure I.8  InVivo HD quadrature extremity coil (GE Healthcare).

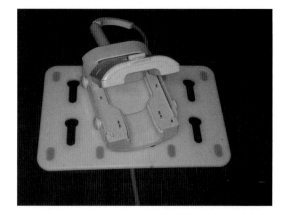

Figure I.10  InVivo 8-channel wrist coil (Philips).

by disease or injury, making it difficult to fit a joint into a coil moulded to the usual body contours.

Small anatomical areas, such as the digits of the hand or foot, require dedicated coils with a small field of view (Fig I.12). Small dual coils are also useful for examination of the temporomandibular joints using a frame to support the coils (Fig I.13).

Imaging coils of the shoulder have possibly the greatest variation in design (Figs I.14–I.16). The coils shown here are merely a sample of the many options available. The coil in Figure I.16 may also be used for imaging of other joints, including the hip and elbow.

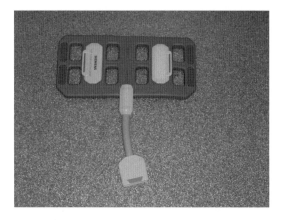

Figure I.11  4-channel small flex coil (Siemens).

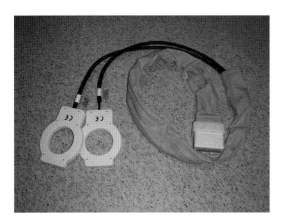

Figure I.12 Three-inch dual coils (GE Healthcare).

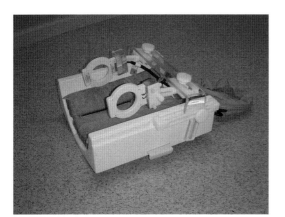

Figure I.13 Three-inch dual coils (GE Healthcare).

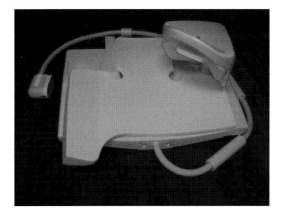

Figure I.14 Shoulder coil (Philips).

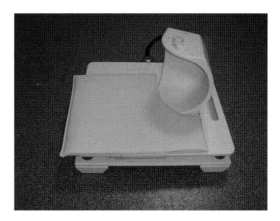

Figure I.15 Shoulder coil (Siemens).

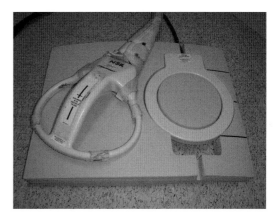

Figure I.16 Multi-purpose phased array coil (MEDRAD).

A specialised coil may be used for imaging of anatomy deep within the pelvis. Such intracavity coils (Fig I.17) provide a small field of view and high signal of structures close to the receiver, such as the prostate, rectum, uterus and anal sphincters. Coils are generally moulded for the particular region of interest; a rectal coil will sit above the sphincters and is therefore not ideal for imaging of the anal sphincters. These coils may often be coupled with other external coils such as that in Figure I.3, and are disposed of once the examination is complete.

Knowing the characteristics of the radiofrequency coil being used and the degree of coverage required

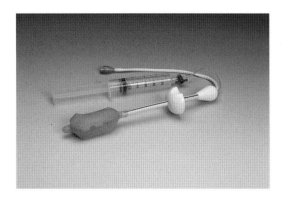

Figure I.17 Endorectal coil MRI probe for prostate (MEDRAD).

for the area and pathology under examination is crucial to producing images of high signal quality. Time spent learning about imaging coil hardware from texts and papers on this subject will be rewarded with comprehension that will enable the radiographer to resolve many issues due to artefacts, save time and generate images of high spatial and contrast resolution.

# Suggested support resources

The websites listed here are of long standing, high repute and hence unlikely to cease to exist in the near future. They offer support to those working with MRI throughout the world, regardless of their specific discipline. All websites were accessible on 14 March 2011.

### Section for Magnetic Resonance Technologists

With chapters in the Australia–New Zealand and Belgium–Netherlands regions as well as across the United States, the Society for Magnetic Resonance Technologists (SMRT) has supported MR radiographers throughout the world for twenty years. With the quarterly Educational Seminars, regional meetings, annual international conference held in conjunction with the International Society for Magnetic Resonance in Medicine (ISMRM), and the associated journals, this organisation provides the widest possible range of educational resources available to the greatest number of people. Make use of the resources on offer and your membership fees will be more than well rewarded.

http://www.ismrm.org/smrt/

### MRI List Server

Free to members and non-members alike, this mail server operated and maintained by the Section for Magnetic Resonance Technologists (SMRT) provides contact with other MR imaging professionals throughout the world. The cumulative body of knowledge of the individuals in this group represents an enormous resource that has assisted and enabled the sharing of information in a bipartisan manner for over a decade.

http://www.ismrm.org/smrt/listserv.htm

### Society for Cardiovascular Magnetic Resonance

Specifically for those involved in cardiovascular MRI. This site provides much support for both members and non-members alike, although some resources require membership.

http://www.scmr.org/

### MRIsafety.com

Set up and maintained by Dr Frank Shellock, this website is invaluable for quickly identifying implant particulars.

http://www.mrisafety.com

### The Adelaide MRI website

Created and maintained by Greg Brown, this resource provides a wealth of information for the MR radiographer. It has been an invaluable tool for countless radiographers over the years and is a useful first port of call for any technical or practical concern.

http://www.users.on.net/~vision/

# Abbreviations

| | |
|---|---|
| ABER | arm abducted and externally rotated |
| ACC | adrenocortical carcinoma |
| ACL | anterior cruciate ligament |
| ACTH | adrenocorticotropic hormone |
| ADIR | arm abducted and internally rotated |
| ALPSA | anterior labroligamentous periosteal sleeve avulsion |
| ASIS | anterior superior iliac spine |
| ATT | anterior tibial tendon |
| AVM | arteriovenous malformation |
| BPH | benign prostatic hyperplasia |
| CBD | common bile duct |
| CLPM | condyle lateral-pterygoid muscle |
| CN | cranial nerve |
| CPA | cerebellopontine angles |
| CSF | cerebrospinal fluid |
| CT | computerised tomography |
| CTN or STN | classic or structural trigeminal neuralgia |
| DRUJ | distal radio-ulnar joint |
| ECG | electrocardiogram or electrocardiograph |
| ERCP | endoscopic retrograde cholangiopancreatograhpy |
| FABS | flexion and abduction in supination |
| FAI | femoro-acetabular impingement |
| FDL | flexor digitorum longus |
| FHL | flexor hallucis longus |
| FNH | follicular nodular hyperplasia |
| GBM | glioblastoma multiforme |
| GRE | gradient echo |
| HAGL | humeral avulsion glenoid ligament |
| HCC | hepatocellular carcinoma |
| IAC | internal auditory canal |
| IV | intravenous |
| IVC | inferior vena cava |
| LCL | lateral collateral ligament |
| LPM | lateral pterygoid muscle |
| LVLA | left ventricle and left atrium |
| LVOT | left ventricular outflow tract |
| MCL | medial collateral ligament |
| MFH | malignant fibrous histiocytoma |
| MIP | maximum intensity projection |
| MR | magnetic resonance |
| MRA | magnetic resonance angiography |
| MRCP | magnetic resonance cholangiopancreatography |
| MRI | magnetic resonance imaging |
| MS | multiple sclerosis |
| NOF | neck of femur |
| NPC | nasopharyngeal carcinoma |
| OA | osteoarthritis |
| PCC | pheochromocytoma |
| PCL | posterior cruciate ligament |
| PFD | pelvic floor dysfunction |
| PTT | posterior tibial tendon |
| PVNS | pigmented villonodular synovitis |
| RA | rheumatoid arthritis |
| RARE | rapid acquisition and relaxation enhancement |
| RCC | renal cell carcinoma |
| REZ | root exit zone |
| RF | radiofreqency |
| RVOT | right ventricular outflow tract |
| SCC | squamous cell carcinoma |
| SL | scapholunate |
| SLAP | superior labral anterior posterior |
| SNHL | sensorineural hearing loss |
| SOC | synovial osteochondromatosis |
| SOL | space occupying lesion |
| SSFP | single shot fast spin echo |
| SSNHL | sudden sensorineural hearing loss |
| SST | supraspinatous tendon |
| TFCC | triangular fibrocartilage complex injury |
| TMJ | temporomandibular joint |

# Foreword

It is a great pleasure for me to commend this practical book *Planning and Positioning in MRI*. How many MR radiographers have been handed a referral requesting imaging of some part of the body that we have rarely, if ever, had to examine? A text such as this one provides a quick and easy reference to scan positioning.

Anne Bright is a well-known member of the ANZ MR community, both as a member of the Section for Magnetic Resonance Technologists (SMRT) and through having practised in the field of MRI for over fifteen years. In 2002 Anne was awarded Level Two Accreditation with the Australian Institute of Radiography and has maintained her skills to be re-accredited each triennium. *Planning and Positioning in MRI* was researched and written while she was manager of the 1.5 T and 3 T magnets at North Shore Radiology and Nuclear Medicine, within the premises of the North Shore Private Hospital, a site that performs a wide range of MRI examinations for both clinical and research purposes. Recently Anne has moved onto new challenges, establishing a new site and training a new team of staff at Superscan in Parramatta.

When I first met Anne at the combined SMRT/ISMRM conference in Seattle in 2006, she expressed an interest in deepening her involvement in the field of MRI and a desire to make a contribution to the MR community. This book is a testament to her efforts and the experience she has gained in a long and diverse career as an MR Radiographer.

The intent that underpins *Planning and Positioning in MRI* is to assist the practitioner in developing good principles in determining precise image orientation and alignment. In her own role as a manager, Anne observed the relative paucity of information guiding those new to MRI in planning scans.

Relatively few journal articles detail the precise anatomical alignment or coverage when scanning. Discussions with colleagues reinforced her belief that there was a need for a comprehensive guide to scan set-up.

Some may argue that this text is focused too narrowly, with no attention paid to imaging parameters and other technical aspects associated with planning an MR scan. That information is available to the reader through an extensive array of textbooks already on the market and would have proven too burdensome to add to this text. Instead what we have is a dedicated text focused solely on scan set-up. *Planning and Positioning in MRI* serves the purpose for our industry that a basic radiography positioning text provides the general radiographer. The case studies provided on the associated website give a brief overview of the interplay of image orientation with the parameter selection. Their intention is to prompt the practitioner to think about the many variables inherent in image planning, of which scan orientation is but one, and to assist the practitioner in developing an effective thought process for examination workflow.

*Planning and Positioning in MRI* will be a valuable source of practical information for students and beginners, and also a useful reference text for those more experienced. I recommend it as a reference text that should be available in all clinical MR centres.

Wendy Strugnell BAppSc (MIT)
Director of MRI Services, The Prince Charles
Hospital, Brisbane, Australia
Past President 2008–2009, Section for Magnetic
Resonance Technologists of the International
Society of Magnetic Resonance in Medicine

# Acknowledgements

A team of people, both personal and professional, has supported me. Without them this tome may not have been realised.

First Luisa Cecotti, who so graciously threw me off the cliff when I was too timid to crawl to the edge. Without your push, I would probably still be ruminating about the possibilities.

Sunalie Silva, Melinda McEvoy, Samantha McCulloch, Rebecca Cornell, Natalie Hamad and Helena Klijn at Elsevier and Brenda Hamilton. You kept reassuring me of the efficacy of this project, believing in what I often doubted. Thank you.

My employers at North Shore Radiology have been wildly enthusiastic about my efforts to write this book. Especial thanks must go to Dr James Christie, who provided unfettered access and support for the collection of images and access to literature. In conjunction with Dr David Brazier and Dr Bruno Guiffre, Dr Christie has acted as the source of numerous practical conversations regarding imaging protocols that have translated into material for both this text and the imaging manual within the business itself. I have indeed learned an enormous amount under your tutelage and that of all the radiologists at NSR. It is a privilege to work with you.

Midland MRI in Hamilton, New Zealand kindly provided some of the images used in this text. Dr Glenn Coltman and Stephen Butler shared their knowledge and the company's vast array of images and protocols, particularly for MR angiography. I am immensely grateful for their time, hospitality, opinions and access to their database.

Grateful thanks are due to Dr Iain Duncan and Luke Denyer at the Canberra Imaging Group and to Vanessa Pineiro at PRP Imaging in Gordon, Sydney for allowing me to visit and collect data from their sites. Wendy Strugnell at The Prince Charles Hospital in Brisbane and Dr Gemma Figtree from the Department of Cardiology, Royal North Shore Hospital provided assistance with details in cardiac imaging. Thanks also to Paul Dobie from Radar Imaging in Melbourne.

The MRI radiographers at North Shore Radiology have tolerated my quizzing and assisted in the search for the images that have formed the basis of this text. Thanks Matt Hammond. Let's get those hamstrings to London for 2012!

Thanks to all the vendor representatives who assisted with approval of images of the coils shown, in particular Imbi Semenov, Anne Davidson and Barbara Pirgousis (GE Healthcare); David Kent, Derby Chang, Kathleen Dunst and Timothy Hands (Imaxeon/Medrad); Peter Pasfield (Philips); Wellsley Were, May Teo and Jo Ellerton (Siemens).

In everything we do, family should come first. For me, the effort that has gone into producing this work would be meaningless if those I hold most dear had failed to believe in and support me. No child could have wanted for greater support in pursuing an education than that with which my siblings and I have been blessed by our parents. This is true inheritance.

My brother Neil Bright has shared his considerable knowledge of anatomy and pathology throughout my professional life. All those books and gory images you showed me as a child came to something. At least the rest of the family won't mind me showing them a picture from this one after dinner!

Last, but never, ever the least, to my Wiradjuri Warrior. Our mutual respect and intellectual sparring has fired the motivation behind what was only in its infancy when we first met. Your trust in my abilities gave stability when I felt the task all-consuming and my self-belief wavering. We work so very well together. Whatever challenges and despite the adversities, you always manage to weave with me another line in our cloth. The publication of this book is definitely a golden thread.

# Reviewers

**Clare Berry**
Conjoint Diploma in Diagnostic Radiography,
Postgraduate Certificate in MRI
Royal Brisbane and Women's Hospital,
Queensland University of Technology

**Stephen Butler**
MHSc(MRI), Member SMRT & NZIMRT
Midland MRI, Hamilton, NZ

**Gail Durbridge**
MSc
Senior Research Radiographer
Coordinator MRT Teaching Program,
Centre for Magnetic Resonance,
University of Queensland

**Nicole Harrison**
Bachelor of Medical Radiation Science (Diagnostic
Radiography)
Blacktown / Mt Druitt Hospital, NSW

**Kerri Oshust**
MRT (MR)
Instructor in MRI Program,
School of Health Sciences
Coordinator, MRI Second Discipline,
Department of Continuing Education,
NAIT, Canada

**Mark W Strudwick**
PhD, PGDip Magnetic Resonance Technology, Dip
Diagnostic Radiography
Senior Lecturer,
Dept. of Medical Imaging & Radiation Sciences,
School of Biomedical Sciences,
Faculty of Medicine, Nursing and Health Sciences,
Monash University, Vic.

**Lawrance Yip**
MSc Magnetic Resonance Technology
Department of Radiology, Queen Mary Hospital,
Hong Kong

**Bosco Yu**
Master of Health Science—MRI, Bachelor of
Business, Dip in Law
MRI Portfolio Manager, Blacktown Hospital, NSW
Member of Medical Imaging Advisory Panel,
Australian Institute of Radiography

# Figure and picture credits

Figures I.1, I.4, I.5, I.8, I.12 and I.13: images kindly provided by GE Healthcare. © 2010 GE Healthcare Australia Pty Ltd. All rights reserved.

Figures I.2, I.6, I.9, I.11 and I.15: images kindly provided by Siemens Australia & New Zealand.

Figures I.3, I.7, I.10 and I.14: images kindly provided by Philips Australia.

Figures I.16 and I.17: images kindly provided by MEDRAD Radiology.

Figures 3.53, 3.55, 3.57 and 4.45: images kindly provided by Midland MRI, Hamilton, New Zealand.

All other MR images sourced from North Shore Radiology. Without the support of my employers, North Shore Radiology, Sydney, this book would never have happened, and it showcases the quality of work they produce.

Thanks also to Netter Images (www.netterimages. com © Elsevier Inc.); Drake (*Gray's Anatomy for Students 2e*); Canberra Imaging Group; and PRP Diagnostic Imaging, Gordon, Sydney.

# Section 1

# Head and neck

# Cranial nerves

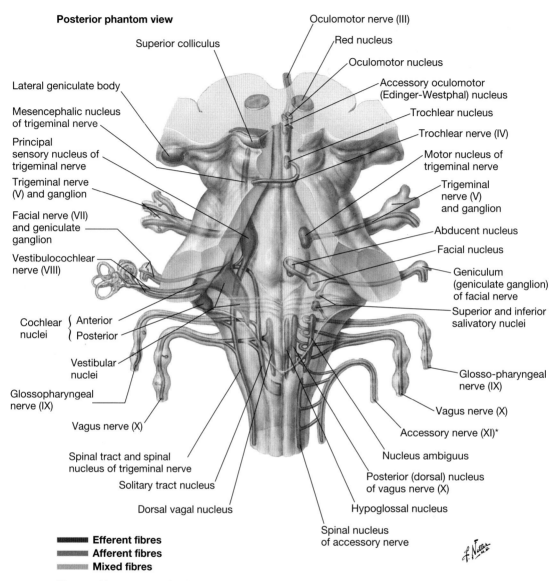

**Efferent fibres**
**Afferent fibres**
**Mixed fibres**

*Recent evidence suggests that the accessory nerve lacks a cranial root and has no connection to the vagus nerve. Verification of this finding awaits further investigation.

Figure 1.1  Coronal brainstem.
(Netter illustration from www.netterimages.com ©Elsevier Inc. All rights reserved.)

# Cranial nerve nuclei in brainstem: schema

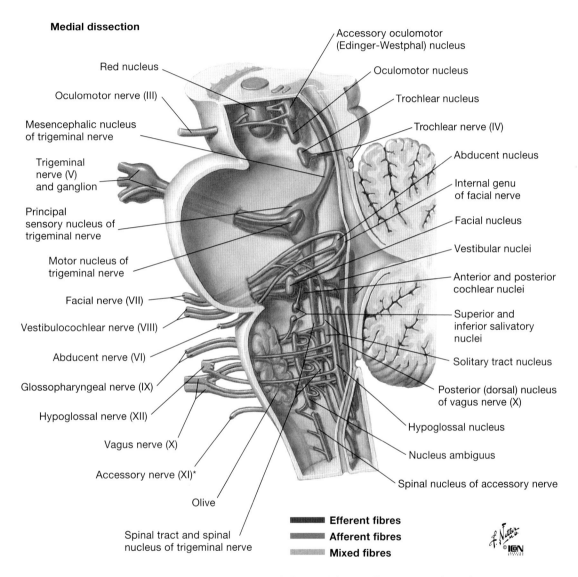

**Medial dissection**

Red nucleus

Oculomotor nerve (III)

Mesencephalic nucleus of trigeminal nerve

Trigeminal nerve (V) and ganglion

Principal sensory nucleus of trigeminal nerve

Motor nucleus of trigeminal nerve

Facial nerve (VII)

Vestibulocochlear nerve (VIII)

Abducent nerve (VI)

Glossopharyngeal nerve (IX)

Hypoglossal nerve (XII)

Vagus nerve (X)

Accessory nerve (XI)*

Olive

Spinal tract and spinal nucleus of trigeminal nerve

Accessory oculomotor (Edinger-Westphal) nucleus

Oculomotor nucleus

Trochlear nucleus

Trochlear nerve (IV)

Abducent nucleus

Internal genu of facial nerve

Facial nucleus

Vestibular nuclei

Anterior and posterior cochlear nuclei

Superior and inferior salivatory nuclei

Solitary tract nucleus

Posterior (dorsal) nucleus of vagus nerve (X)

Hypoglossal nucleus

Nucleus ambiguus

Spinal nucleus of accessory nerve

Efferent fibres
Afferent fibres
Mixed fibres

*Recent evidence suggests that the accessory nerve lacks a cranial root and has no connection to the vagus nerve. Verification of this finding awaits further investigation

Figure 1.2 Sagittal brainstem.

# Cranial nerves: names and numbering

| I | Olfactory | VII | Facial |
|---|-----------|-----|--------|
| II | Optic | VIII | Vestibulocochlear |
| III | Oculomotor | IX | Glossopharyngeal |
| IV | Trochlear | X | Vagus |
| V | Trigeminal | XI | Accessory |
| VI | Abducent | XII | Hypoglossal |

# Chapter 1.1 Brain

## Indications:

- Headache
- Space occupying lesion (SOL) or tumour, e.g. meningioma, astrocytoma, glioblastoma multiforme (GBM), metastases
- Generalised non-specific symptoms
- Arachnoid cyst
- Demyelination, e.g. multiple sclerosis (MS)
- Stroke, vertigo
- Epidermoid
- Encephalitis or meningitis
- Arteriovenous malformation (AVM)
- Seizure.

**Cerebrum: medial views**

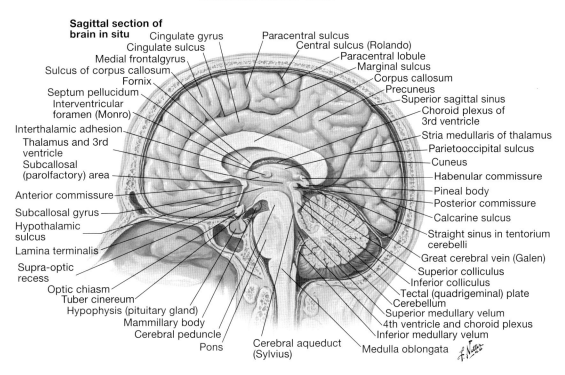

Figure 1.3 Mid-sagittal section through the brain.
(Netter illustration from www.netterimages.com ©Elsevier Inc. All rights reserved.)

## Coils and patient considerations

Contained within the cranial vault, the brain is subject to a myriad of pathological conditions. Patients who present with vague symptoms affecting multiple bodily functions, with systemic disease or suggestive of vascular compromise often require imaging of the entire brain to determine disease extent, before proceeding with a more targeted examination.

Commencing inferiorly the cervical portion of the spinal cord meets with the brainstem, formed by the medulla oblongata, pons and midbrain. Posterior to the brainstem, the cerebellum is separated by the fourth ventricle. Cerebrospinal fluid (CSF) passes through the cerebral aqueduct into the third ventricle, located between the thalami. The foramina of Monro allow CSF to communicate with the lateral ventricles. The anterior horn of each lateral ventricle resides in the frontal lobe, the posterior horns in the occipital lobes and the inferior horns in the temporal lobes.

Scanning a routine 'bulk standard' protocol will not suffice for all cases, however for many the imaging coil of choice will not vary. A dedicated head coil (Fig 1.6, shown with neck elements attached) is preferred for examination solely of the brain. Some coils are scalable, allowing additional components to be attached, increasing anatomical coverage (Figs 1.4, 1.5 & 1.6). There are occasions when only a transmit–receive coil may be used, most notably when imaging patients with deep brain stimulators in situ. Significant safety concerns exist in this type of scenario so the reader is strongly advised to thoroughly research these issues with the implant manufacturer and the many safety resources and articles available both locally and internationally prior to proceeding.

Kyphotic patients may not be able to tilt the head forward to enable the head to fit within the coil with ease. Placing pillows or cushions beneath the patient's buttocks may ameliorate this problem, reducing the degree of extension between the head and neck so that the chin is lowered within the coil. Extra padding beneath the knees may be required to make this position tolerable.

# Imaging planes: Routine sequences

## Position:

- Supine, head first.

## Other considerations:

- The patient should be well padded to prevent image degradation or malalignment due to head movement.
- If the imaging coil has a mirror, ensure the patient is able to see out of the bore to alleviate claustrophobia.
- Orientation of axial images may vary between sites. An alternate orientation is aligned to the hard palate. This is a highly site-specific issue and the radiographer should adhere to the site protocol; variation in alignment between time points may complicate and limit ability to determine disease variation, especially when measuring mass lesions.

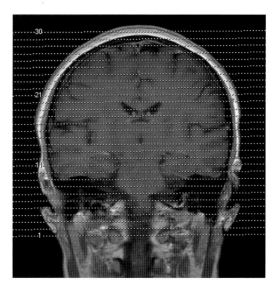

Figure 1.5 Axial planning on a coronal image. (North Shore Radiology)

## Axial

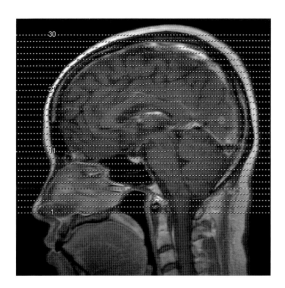

Figure 1.4 Axial planning on a sagittal image. (North Shore Radiology)

## Alignment:

- Parallel to a line joining the splenium and genu of the corpus callosum (sub callosal line).

## Coverage:

*Superior to inferior:*
- Craniocervical junction to vertex

*Lateral to medial:*
- Temporal lobes on both sides

*Posterior to anterior:*
- Occipital to frontal lobes.

## Demonstrates:

- Midline shift caused by a SOL
- Ventricular dimensions and asymmetry
- Asymmetry of the cerebellar or cerebral hemispheres
- Origins of the cranial nerves.

# Coronal

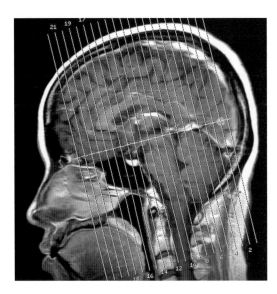

Figure 1.6 Coronal planning on a sagittal image.
(North Shore Radiology)

## Alignment:

· Parallel to the brainstem.

## Coverage:

*Superior to inferior:*
· Craniocervical junction to vertex

*Lateral to medial:*
· Temporal lobes on both sides

*Posterior to anterior:*
· Occipital to frontal lobes.

## Demonstrates:

· As per axial oblique plane
· Best plane for demonstrating lesions superior to the cribriform plate
· Masses in the brainstem and origins of the cranial nerves.

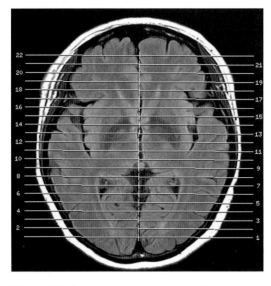

Figure 1.7 Coronal planning on an axial image.
(North Shore Radiology)

# Sagittal

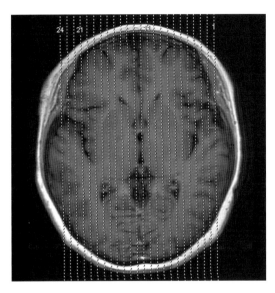

Figure 1.8 Sagittal planning on an axial image.
(North Shore Radiology)

## Alignment:

- Parallel to the falx
- If midline shift is evident, a line of best fit should be used.

## Coverage:

*Superior to inferior:*
- Craniocervical junction to vertex

*Lateral to medial:*
- Temporal lobes on each side

*Posterior to anterior:*
- Occipital to frontal lobes.

## Demonstrates:

- Brainstem compression or Arnold-Chiari malformation
- Craniocervical lesions
- Masses in the frontal fossa +/− breach of the cribriform plate
- Partial or total agenesis of the corpus callosum.

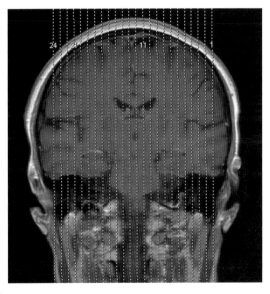

Figure 1.9 Sagittal planning on a coronal image.
(North Shore Radiology)

# Chapter 1.2 Pituitary

## Indications:

- Macroadenoma
- Microadenoma or prolactinoma
- Delayed onset or precocious puberty
- Galactorrhoea
- Menstrual irregularity or amenorrhoea
- Bitemporal hemianopia (loss of the lateral half of the visual field in both eyes, with sparing of medial vision)
- Cushing's disease (ACTH dependent Cushing's syndrome)
- Rathke's cleft cyst
- Craniopharyngioma
- Diabetes insipidus
- Pituitary apoplexy (due to infarction or haemorrhage).

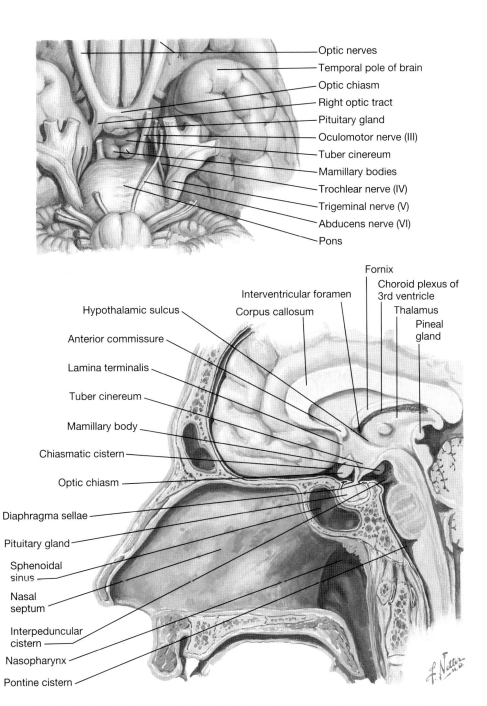

Optic nerves
Temporal pole of brain
Optic chiasm
Right optic tract
Pituitary gland
Oculomotor nerve (III)
Tuber cinereum
Mamillary bodies
Trochlear nerve (IV)
Trigeminal nerve (V)
Abducens nerve (VI)
Pons

Fornix
Choroid plexus of
3rd ventricle
Thalamus
Pineal
gland

Interventricular foramen
Corpus callosum

Hypothalamic sulcus
Anterior commissure
Lamina terminalis
Tuber cinereum
Mamillary body
Chiasmatic cistern
Optic chiasm
Diaphragma sellae
Pituitary gland
Sphenoidal
sinus
Nasal
septum
Interpeduncular
cistern
Nasopharynx
Pontine cistern

Figure 1.10 Relationship of the pituitary gland to the brain, optic nerves and cavernous sinus (A).
(Netter illustration from www.netterimages.com ©Elsevier Inc. All rights reserved.)

http://evolve.elsevier.com/AU/Bright/positioning/

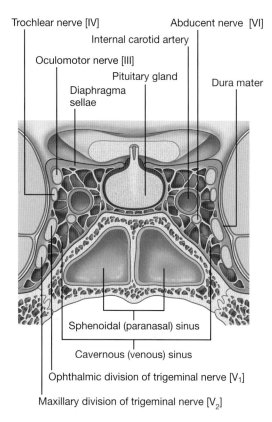

Trochlear nerve [IV]

Abducent nerve  [VI]

Internal carotid artery

Oculomotor nerve [III]

Pituitary gland

Diaphragma
sellae

Dura mater

Sphenoidal (paranasal) sinus

Cavernous (venous) sinus

Ophthalmic division of trigeminal nerve [V₁]

Maxillary division of trigeminal nerve [V₂]

Figure 1.11 Relationship of the pituitary gland to
the brain and cavernous sinus (B).
(From Drake, Gray's Anatomy for Students 2e, with
permission)

## Coils and patient considerations

Sitting within the sella turcica of the sphenoid bone immediately superior to the sphenoid sinus is the pituitary gland (also known as the hypophysis). Outside the blood–brain barrier, but still encased within the dura, the pituitary is the 'control centre' for the other endocrine organs of the body.

The neurohypophysis (posterior lobe) is separated from the adenohypophysis (anterior lobe) by the intermediate lobe (pars intermedius). Rising superiorly from the neurohypophysis, the infundibulum connects the gland with the hypothalamus superiorly and immediately posterior to the optic chiasm. The cavernous sinus, containing the siphon of the internal carotid artery and cranial nerves III, IV and V, is found laterally on each side. The clinoid processes of the sella form the anterior and posterior bony boundaries. The lack of a bony boundary lateral to the pituitary makes lesion expansion into the cavernous sinus a not infrequent consequence of disease.

Lesions of the pituitary vary dramatically in size. Microadenomas are defined as being less than 10 mm in diameter. Larger lesions, such as macroadenomas and craniopharyngiomas, may induce pressure on the optic chiasm resulting in visual disturbance and headaches. A survey of the whole brain in the axial plane as described in Chapter 1.1 can be useful in providing an overview of the extent of disease before planning the more specific planes listed in this section. Planning to cover just between the anterior and posterior clinoid processes may be insufficient and consideration must always be given to increasing coverage should pathology extend beyond the boundaries prescribed in the following plans.

The same imaging coil and patient considerations described in Chapter 1.1 should be applied for examination of the pituitary.

# Imaging planes: Routine sequences

## Position:

- Supine, head first.

## Other considerations:

- The patient should be well padded to prevent image degradation or malalignment due to head movement.
- If the imaging coil has a mirror, ensure the patient is able to see out of the bore to alleviate claustrophobia.

## Sagittal

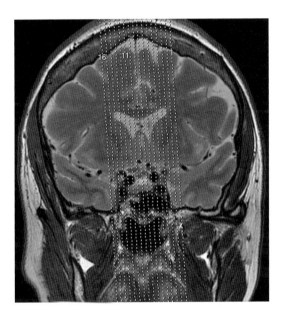

**Figure 1.12** Sagittal planning on a coronal image. (North Shore Radiology)

## Alignment:

- Parallel to the falx in both the coronal and sagittal planes.

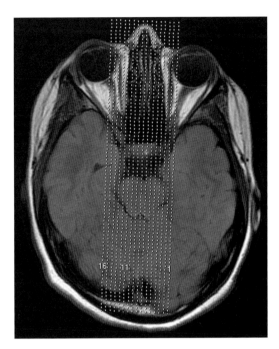

**Figure 1.13** Sagittal planning on an axial image. (North Shore Radiology)

## Coverage:

*Superior to inferior:*
- Floor of the sphenoid sinus to the genu of the corpus callosum

*Lateral to medial:*
- Cavernous sinus on each side

*Posterior to anterior:*
- Ventral aspect of the pons to the anterior clinoid process.

## Demonstrates:

- Elevation of the optic chiasm by a mass within the sella turcica
- Lesion invasion of the carotid siphon, sphenoid sinus and/or brainstem
- Pituitary infundibulum connecting the hypothalamus and the posterior pituitary
- Sella thinning, expansion or destruction.

# Coronal

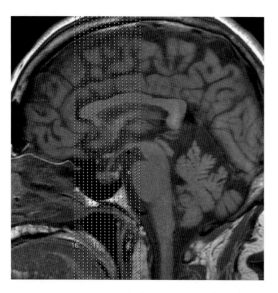

Figure 1.14 Coronal planning on a sagittal image. (North Shore Radiology)

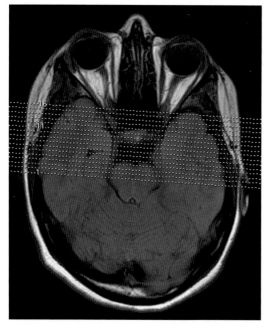

Figure 1.15 Coronal planning on an axial image. (North Shore Radiology)

## Alignment:

- Perpendicular to the floor of the sella on a sagittal image
- Perpendicular to the midline of the brain on an axial image.

## Coverage:

- As for the sagittal plane.

## Demonstrates:

- Elevation of the optic chiasm by a mass within the sella turcica
- Lesion invasion of the carotid siphon, sphenoid sinus and/or brainstem
- Cavernous sinus disruption.

# Chapter 1.3 Orbits (CN II)

## Indications:

- Retro-orbital lesions +/− proptosis
- Optic disc distortion or pallor
- Infection or inflammation, e.g. orbital cellulitis
- Intra-ocular lesions
- Retinoblastoma
- Melanoma
- Orbital infections.

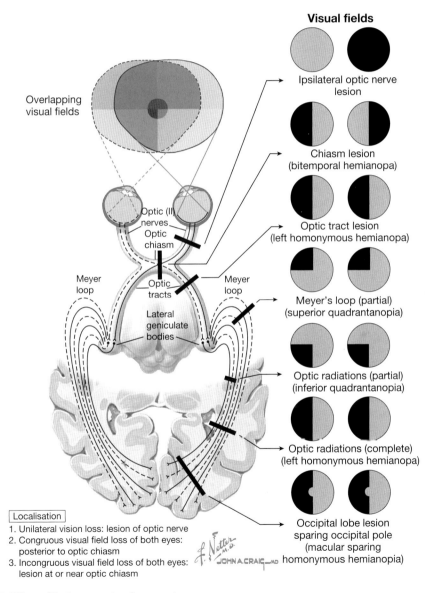

**Visual fields**

Ipsilateral optic nerve lesion

Chiasm lesion (bitemporal hemianopa)

Optic tract lesion (left homonymous hemianopa)

Meyer's loop (partial) (superior quadrantanopia)

Optic radiations (partial) (inferior quadrantanopia)

Optic radiations (complete) (left homonymous hemianopa)

Occipital lobe lesion sparing occipital pole (macular sparing homonymous hemianopia)

Overlapping visual fields

Optic (II) nerves
Optic chiasm

Meyer loop

Optic tracts

Meyer loop

Lateral geniculate bodies

Localisation
1. Unilateral vision loss: lesion of optic nerve
2. Congruous visual field loss of both eyes: posterior to optic chiasm
3. Incongruous visual field loss of both eyes: lesion at or near optic chiasm

**Figure 1.16** Effect of lesions on visual perception.
(Netter illustration from www.netterimages.com ©Elsevier Inc. All rights reserved.)

## Coils and patient considerations

The paired optic nerves (CNII) course from the retina posteromedially to the optic chiasm, immediately superior to the pituitary. Determining the region to examine when a patient has visual loss can be problematic. Figure 1.15 demonstrates the effect of lesions along various portions of the visual pathway. Total visual loss in one eye or bitemporal hemianopia (loss of vision in the lateral half of both eyes) indicates a lesion affecting the chiasm or the nerve between the chiasm and the globe. Beyond the chiasm, examination of the brain is required rather than simply the orbits.

Patients should be asked to close the eyes during image acquisition to limit ocular movement that may degrade image quality. The use of an eye mask may be helpful. Alternately, providing the opportunity to the patient to open the eyes between scans may suffice.

The same imaging coil and patient considerations described in Chapter 1.1 should be applied for examination of the orbits. Sagittal imaging is not a standard requirement but, if required, positioning and planning is as described in Chapter 1.1.

# Imaging planes: Routine sequences

## Position:

- Supine, head first.

## Other considerations:

- The patient should be well padded to prevent image degradation or malalignment due to head movement.
- If the imaging coil has a mirror, ensure the patient is able to see out of the bore to alleviate claustrophobia.

## Axial

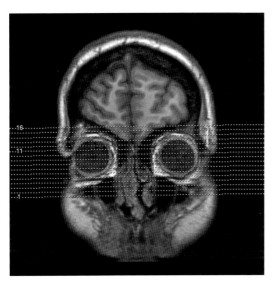

Figure 1.17 Axial planning on a coronal image.
(North Shore Radiology)

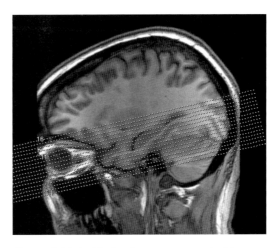

Figure 1.18 Axial planning on a parasagittal image, aligned to the optic nerve.
(North Shore Radiology)

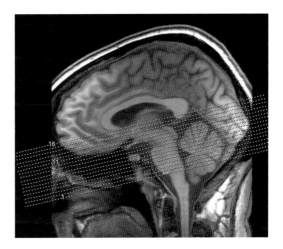

Figure 1.19 Axial planning on a mid-sagittal image.
(North Shore Radiology)

## Alignment:

- Parallel to a line joining the inferior orbital margins
- In-plane with the optic nerve.

## Coverage:

*Superior to inferior:*
- Inferior to superior orbital margin

*Lateral to medial:*
- Zygoma on each side

*Posterior to anterior:*
- Mid pons to anterior aspect of the globes.

## Demonstrates:

- Alignment of the globes and proptosis due to a mass posteriorly
- Disruption of retro-orbital fat
- Optic nerve compression/invasion
- Bony destruction laterally
- The lens between the anterior and posterior chambers and the vitreal chamber posteriorly.

# Coronal

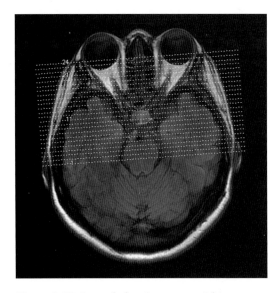

Figure 1.20 Coronal planning on an axial image. (North Shore Radiology)

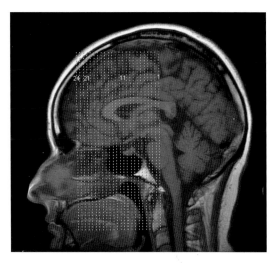

Figure 1.21 Coronal planning on a sagittal image. (North Shore Radiology)

## Alignment:

- Parallel to a line joining the posterior orbital margins
- Perpendicular to the cribriform plate.

## Coverage:

- As per axial scans.

## Demonstrates:

- Disruption of retro-orbital fat
- Optic nerve compression/invasion
- Bony destruction superiorly and inferiorly +/− involvement of the frontal lobe or sinuses
- Passage of the optic nerve from the pons, through the optic foramen to the retina
- Compromise of other structures within the cavernous sinus
- Elevation of the chiasm by a pituitary mass
- Mass within the vitreal chamber.

# Chapter 1.4 Trigeminal nerve (CN V)

ONLINE CASE STUDY
CS5

## Indications:

- Trigeminal neuralgia (tic doloreux) or facial pain +/− facial spasm
  - Classed as 'classic' (CTN) or structural (STN)
- Vascular compression at the root exit zone (REZ; the most common cause of pain)
- Mass, trigeminal schwannoma/neuroma

- Type I neurofibromatosis
- Hamartoma
- Meningioma
- Epidermoid cyst
- Infection
- All the indications in Chapter 1.1.

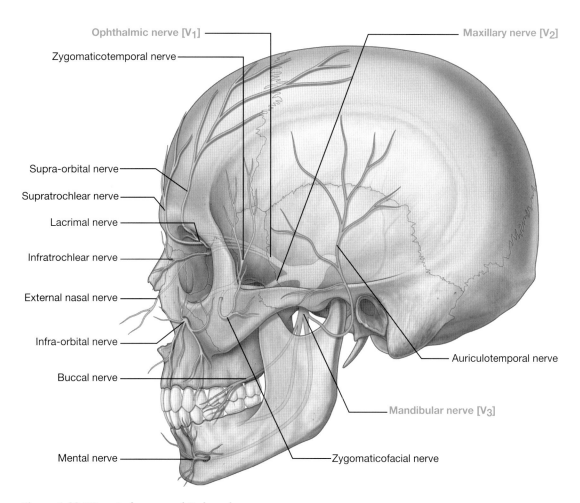

Figure 1.22 Trigeminal nerve and its branches.
(From Drake, Gray's Anatomy for Students 2e, with permission)

# Coils and patient considerations

Originating at the anterolateral aspect of the pons, the trigeminal nerve traverses Meckel's cave posterolateral to the cavernous sinus; this short section is referred to as the root exit zone (REZ). Beyond this CSF-filled space lies the Gasserian ganglion, at which point the nerve branches into its three divisions. The ophthalmic nerve ($V_1$) courses anteriorly from the ganglion through the cavernous sinus to enter the orbit via the superior orbital fissure. The second, maxillary branch ($V_2$), passes through the cavernous sinus and the foramen rotundum before dividing again, the largest branch continuing as the infra-orbital nerve coursing through the orbital floor. The mandibular branch ($V_3$) drops inferiorly without entering the cavernous sinus, exiting the skull at the foramen ovale and dividing within the masticator space. Sensory disturbance may indicate the specific branch suffering disease, but all segments should be included in examination (Fig 1.22).

The trigeminal nerve has an extensive sensory and motor origin within the brainstem and upper cervical cord, reaching from the inferior colliculus to the level of the second cervical vertebra. Hence pathology may originate or extend beyond the nerve itself, such as in syringobulbia (see Ch 2.1 for imaging of a syrinx). Clinically, what may appear to be trigeminal in origin may actually be the result of more diffuse disease or a large mass inducing direct pressure from one of the other cranial nerves, although in such cases the patient would usually exhibit symptoms affecting more than just CN V. Consequently, imaging of the trigeminal nerve should always include imaging of the brain as a whole, ensuring that more extensive disease (e.g. MS or syringomyelia) is fully appreciated.

Vascular anomalies inducing compression at the root exit zone have been argued as a possible aetiology for pain, although not all authors concur. Regardless, a MR angiogram is also often requested. See Chapter 1.12 for scan plans.

The same imaging coil and patient considerations described in Chapter 1.1 should be applied.

# Imaging planes: Routine sequences

## Position:

- Supine, head first.

## Other considerations:

- The patient should be well padded to prevent image degradation or malalignment due to head movement.
- If the imaging coil has a mirror, ensure the patient is able to see out of the bore to alleviate claustrophobia.

## Axial: brainstem

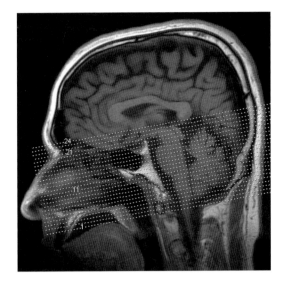

Figure 1.24 Axial planning on a sagittal image.
(North Shore Radiology)

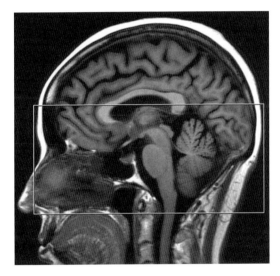

Figure 1.23 Volume acquisition planned axially on a sagittal image.
(North Shore Radiology)

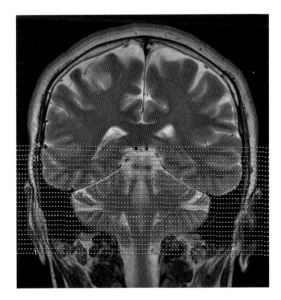

Figure 1.25 Axial planning on a coronal image.
(North Shore Radiology)

## Alignment:

- Perpendicular to the brainstem
- Note that a 3D volume may be planned in a true axial plane and sectioned appropriately as reformats (Fig 1.23).

## Coverage:

*Superior to inferior:*
- Foramen magnum to tectum (corpora quadrigemina)
- If the cerebellar tonsils protrude through the foramen (as with Arnold-Chiari malformation), scans must be extended to ensure complete coverage

*Lateral to medial:*
- Temporal bones on both sides

*Posterior to anterior:*
- Pons to face, including the sinuses and mandible.

## Demonstrates:

- Origin of CN V at the pons and cranial nerves II to XII
- Compression of the REZ by vascular anomalies or lesions of the other cranial nerves
- Masses within Meckel's cave or along the length of the branches
- Sub tentorial masses and compression of posterior cranial structures.

# Coronal

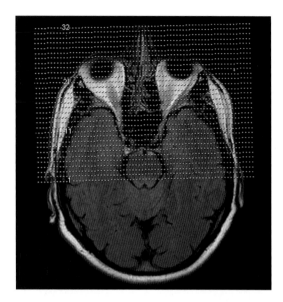

Figure 1.26 Coronal planning on an axial image. (North Shore Radiology)

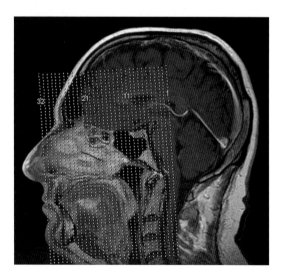

Figure 1.27 Coronal planning on a sagittal image. (North Shore Radiology)

## Alignment:

- Parallel to the brainstem.

## Coverage:

*Superior to inferior:*
- Mandibular ramus to tectum (corpora quadrigemina)

*Lateral to medial:*
- Temporal bones on both sides

*Posterior to anterior:*
- Pons to face, including the sinuses and mandible.

## Demonstrates:

- Compression of the REZ by vascular anomalies or lesions of the other cranial nerves
- Masses within Meckel's cave or the cavernous sinus
- Masses anywhere along the length of any of the branches.

# Axial: nerve roots

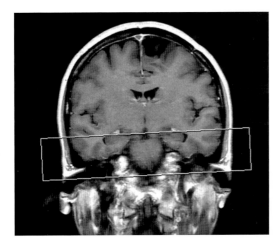

Figure 1.28 Axial volume acquisition targeted to the CN V nerve roots, planned on a coronal image. (North Shore Radiology)

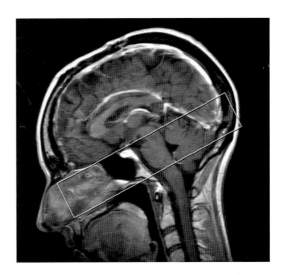

Figure 1.29 Axial volume acquisition targeted to the CN V nerve roots, planned on a sagittal image. (North Shore Radiology)

## Alignment:

- Perpendicular to the brainstem.

## Coverage:

*Superior to inferior:*
- Entire pons

*Lateral to medial:*
- Full width of the brainstem

*Posterior to anterior:*
- Pons to the face.

## Demonstrates:

- Origin of the nerve at the pons and REZ
- Compression by masses or vessels.

# Chapter 1.5 Cerebellopontine angles (CN VII–VIII)

## Indications:

- Sensorineural hearing loss (SNHL), possibly sudden (SSNHL)
- Conductive hearing loss
- Sudden or fluctuating hearing loss
- Acoustic schwannoma (neuroma)
- Constant or pulsatile tinnitus (the latter may be indicative of vascular compression, malformation or glomus jugulare; see Ch 1.6)
- Vertigo, disequilibrium or Meniere's disease
- Vascular compression at the root exit zone
- Type 2 neurofibromatosis (associated with bilateral acoustic schwannomas)
- Facial numbness or weakness
- Known CPA lesion or schwannoma +/− hydrocephalus
- Infection, e.g. Bell's palsy
- First branchial cleft cyst.

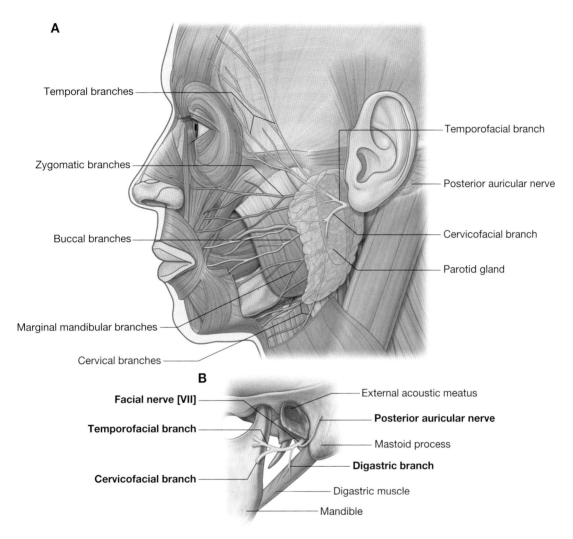

Figure 1.30 Cranial nerve VII and its branches.
(From Drake, Gray's Anatomy for Students 2e, with permission)

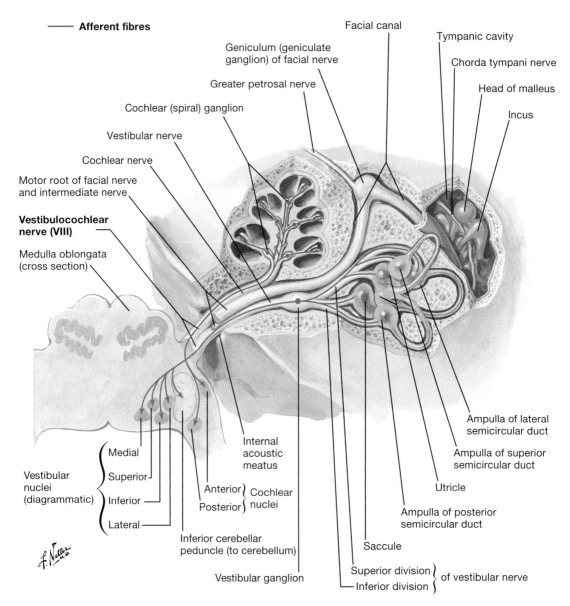

Figure 1.31  Cranial nerve VIII.
(Netter illustration from www.netterimages.com ©Elsevier Inc. All rights reserved.)

# Coils and patient considerations

Bounded by the brainstem medially, cerebellum superoposteriorly, temporal bone laterally and the arachnoid covering of cranial nerves (CN) IX to XII inferiorly, the cerebellopontine angles (CPA) form the CSF-filled spaces through which the facial (VII) and vestibulocochlear (VIII) nerves course before entering the internal auditory canal (IAC). CSF within the canals is continuous with the CPA. Cranial nerve VII originates medially from the pons slightly superoanterior to CN VIII. In the distal portion of the IAC the eighth cranial nerve divides into vestibular and cochlear branches; the vestibular nerve divides more distally, producing an inferior and superior branch (Fig 1.31). The total distance from the origin of CN VIII to its branches is approximately 25 mm.

Lesions that extend peripherally along the labyrinthine branch of CN VII are usually facial in origin, particularly if a 'tail' is evident and there is invasion of the geniculate ganglion. The Schwann cell sheath surrounding the facial nerve begins soon after it exits the pons within the CPA, unlike that of the vestibulocochlear nerve, which commences just before entering the IAC; until this point it is surrounded by oligodendroglia. Consequently, acoustic schwannomas generally originate within the IAC, most commonly on the vestibular division, extruding medially into the CPA with increased size. Tumours that do not obviously originate within the canal and compress the midbrain are unlikely to be of acoustic origin, and may require imaging of a larger portion of the midbrain and post fossa than simply the IACs. Those presenting with large lesions may suffer headaches due to distortion of the fourth ventricle. Such large masses may require extra imaging of the posterior fossa as set out in Chapter 1.6.

Clinical differentiation between potential lesions of CN V and CN VII can be difficult as there is overlap in the regions innervated (compare Figs 1.22 & 1.30). Requests to image patients presenting with facial symptoms may need to be reviewed by a radiologist to ensure the correct examination is performed.

In addition, patients with pulsatile tinnitus (as opposed to a constant 'ringing') require a MR angiogram as part of the imaging protocol. Vascular compression of CN VIII is more likely to be responsible for such symptoms than a vestibular schwannoma. See Chapter 1.12 for further information.

The same imaging coil and patient considerations described in Chapter 1.1 should be applied.

# Imaging planes: Routine sequences

## Position:

- Supine, head first.

## Other considerations:

- The patient should be well padded to prevent image degradation or malalignment due to head movement.
- If the imaging coil has a mirror, ensure the patient is able to see out of the bore to alleviate claustrophobia.

## Axial: CPA

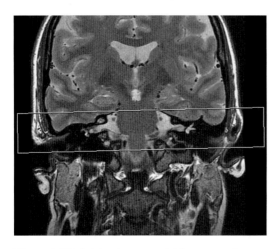

**Figure 1.32** Axial volume acquisition targeted to the CPA, planned on a coronal image.
(North Shore Radiology)

## Alignment:

- Parallel to a line bisecting both IACs.
- Perpendicular to the brainstem in the sagittal plane.
- A 3D volume acquisition is demonstrated above; alignment for a 2D volume would be similar.

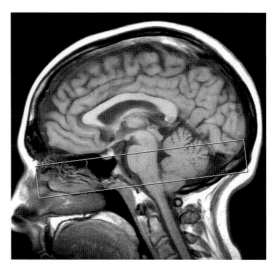

**Figure 1.33** Axial volume acquisition targeted to the CPA, planned on a sagittal image.
(North Shore Radiology)

## Coverage:

*Superior to inferior:*
- Entire CPA
- If a large lesion is evident, extra scans of the posterior fossa may be required to ensure complete coverage

*Lateral to medial:*
- Temporal bones on both sides

*Posterior to anterior:*
- Midbrain to cavernous sinus.

## Demonstrates:

- Origin and divisions of CN VII and VIII
- Compression of the REZ by vascular anomalies or lesions of the other cranial nerves
- Masses within the IACs or their branches.

# Coronal: CPA

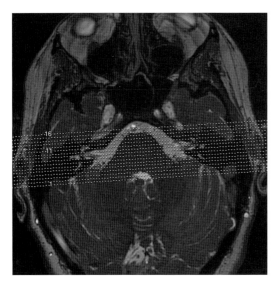

**Figure 1.34** Coronal planning on a sagittal image. (North Shore Radiology)

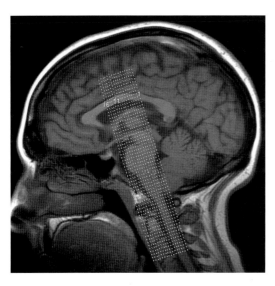

**Figure 1.35** Coronal planning on an axial image. (North Shore Radiology)

## Alignment:

- Parallel to a line bisecting both IACs
- Parallel to the brainstem in the sagittal plane.

## Coverage:

*Superior to inferior:*
- Foramen magnum to the midbrain

*Lateral to medial:*
- Temporal bones on both sides

*Posterior to anterior:*
- Anterior surface of the cerebellum to the anterior aspect of the midbrain.

## Demonstrates:

- Origin and divisions of CN VII and VIII
- Compression of the REZ by vascular anomalies or lesions of the other cranial nerves
- Masses within the IACs or their branches.

# Chapter 1.6 Posterior fossa (CN IX–XII)

## Indications:

- Mass within the posterior fossa, e.g.
  meningioma, epidermoid
- Hydrocephalus
- Glomus tumour or glomus jugulare tumour
  (causing paresis of CN IX–XI)

- Arnold-Chiari malformation
- Perineural invasion from malignancies of the
  nasopharynx.

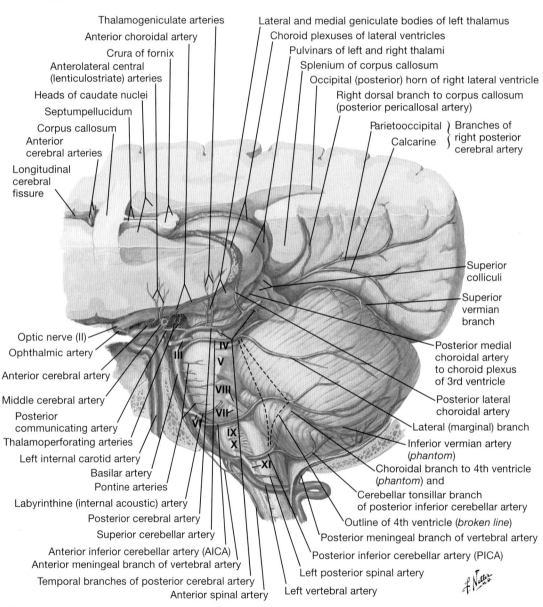

Thalamogeniculate arteries
Anterior choroidal artery
Crura of fornix
Anterolateral central
(lenticulostriate) arteries
Heads of caudate nuclei
Septumpellucidum
Corpus callosum
Anterior
cerebral arteries
Longitudinal
cerebral
fissure

Lateral and medial geniculate bodies of left thalamus
Choroid plexuses of lateral ventricles
Pulvinars of left and right thalami
Splenium of corpus callosum
Occipital (posterior) horn of right lateral ventricle
Right dorsal branch to corpus callosum
(posterior pericallosal artery)
Parietooccipital ⎫ Branches of
           ⎬ right posterior
Calcarine  ⎭ cerebral artery

Superior
colliculi
Superior
vermian
branch

Optic nerve (II)
Ophthalmic artery
Anterior cerebral artery
Middle cerebral artery
Posterior
communicating artery
Thalamoperforating arteries
Left internal carotid artery
Basilar artery
Pontine arteries
Labyrinthine (internal acoustic) artery
Posterior cerebral artery
Superior cerebellar artery
Anterior inferior cerebellar artery (AICA)
Anterior meningeal branch of vertebral artery
Temporal branches of posterior cerebral artery
Anterior spinal artery

III
IV
V
VIII
VII
VI
IX
X
XI

Posterior medial
choroidal artery
to choroid plexus
of 3rd ventricle
Posterior lateral
choroidal artery
Lateral (marginal) branch
Inferior vermian artery
(phantom)
Choroidal branch to 4th ventricle
(phantom) and
Cerebellar tonsillar branch
of posterior inferior cerebellar artery
Outline of 4th ventricle (broken line)
Posterior meningeal branch of vertebral artery
Posterior inferior cerebellar artery (PICA)
Left posterior spinal artery
Left vertebral artery

Figure 1.36 Parasagittal section, demonstrating the anatomy and arteries of the posterior fossa.
(Netter illustration from www.netterimages.com ©Elsevier Inc. All rights reserved.)

# Coils and patient considerations

Imaging of the posterior fossa may be required as part of the examination of cranial nerve pathology. Large lesions within the brainstem or below the tentorium may compress any of cranial nerves III–XII, inducing specific cranial nerve dysfunction or more generalised symptoms. This should always be borne in mind when examining any of the cranial nerves. As CN I and II do not originate within the brainstem more focused attention on the fronto-temporal regions is required, such as for the orbits (Ch 1.3).

The points of origin and manner in which nerves exit the brainstem on each side is often asymmetrical, so alignment of scan planes in the posterior fossa is generally made to the brainstem rather than the individual nerves. Cranial nerves III, IV and VI (oculomotor, trochlear and abducent respectively) and CN $V_1$ and $V_2$ (ophthalmic and maxillary nerves) proceed from the brainstem through the cavernous sinus along with the internal carotid artery. All three nerves continue anteriorly to innervate the muscles of the eye after passing through the superior orbital fissure. Notably, CN IV is the only cranial nerve to originate from the dorsal aspect of the brainstem. Care must be taken when planning coronal scans to ensure that the most posterior portion of this nerve is not missed.

Cranial nerves XI–XII all remain within the posterior fossa until they exit the cranium. The glossopharyngeal and vagus nerves (CN IX and X respectively) originate in the medulla oblongata and exit the skull via the jugular foramen. The spinal accessory nerve originates mainly in the upper spinal cord, ascending through the foramen magnum to merge with fibres of the cranial accessory nerve from the medulla oblongata to form the accessory nerve (CN XI). Most inferiorly is the hypoglossal nerve (CN XII), coursing between the internal carotid artery and the jugular vein before exiting the cranium via the hypoglossal canal, between the foramen magnum and the jugular canal.

The same imaging coil and patient considerations described in Chapter 1.1 should be applied.

# Imaging planes: Routine sequences

## Position:

- Supine, head first.

## Other considerations:

- The patient should be well padded to prevent image degradation or malalignment due to head movement.
- If the imaging coil has a mirror, ensure the patient is able to see out of the bore to alleviate claustrophobia.

# Axial: brainstem

For alignment see Chapter 1.4, Figures 1.23 to 1.25.

## Alignment:

- Aligned perpendicular to the brainstem.
- Note that a 3D volume may be planned in a true axial plane and sectioned appropriately as reformats (Fig 1.23).

## Coverage:

*Superior to inferior:*
- Foramen magnum to tectum (corpora quadrigemina)
- If the cerebellar tonsils protrude through the foramen (as with Arnold-Chiari malformation), scans must be extended to ensure complete coverage

*Lateral to medial:*
- Temporal bones on both sides

*Posterior to anterior:*
- Entire cerebellum and brainstem.

## Demonstrates:

- Origin of cranial nerves II to XII
- Sub tentorial masses and any compression of posterior cranial structures.

# Coronal

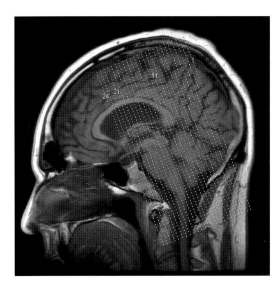

**Figure 1.37** Coronal planning on a sagittal image.
(North Shore Radiology)

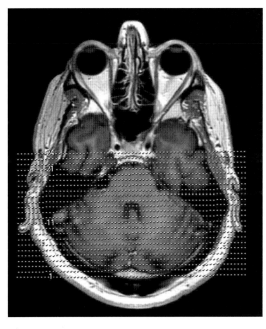

**Figure 1.38** Coronal planning on an axial image.
(North Shore Radiology)

## Alignment:

- Parallel to the brainstem.

## Coverage:

*Superior to inferior:*
- Foramen magnum to splenium of the inferior aspect of the thalamus

*Lateral to medial:*
- Temporal bones on both sides

*Posterior to anterior:*
- Sagittal sinus to posterior clinoids.

## Coverage:

As for the axial plane.

## Demonstrates:

- Origins cranial nerves III to XII
- Sub tentorial masses.

# Chapter 1.7 Temporal lobes

## Indications:

- Epilepsy or first seizure (simple partial or complex seizures)
- Mesial temporal sclerosis
- EEG abnormality

- Abnormal grey matter migration
- Assessment of hippocampal volume
- Sensations of déjà vu or jamais vu.

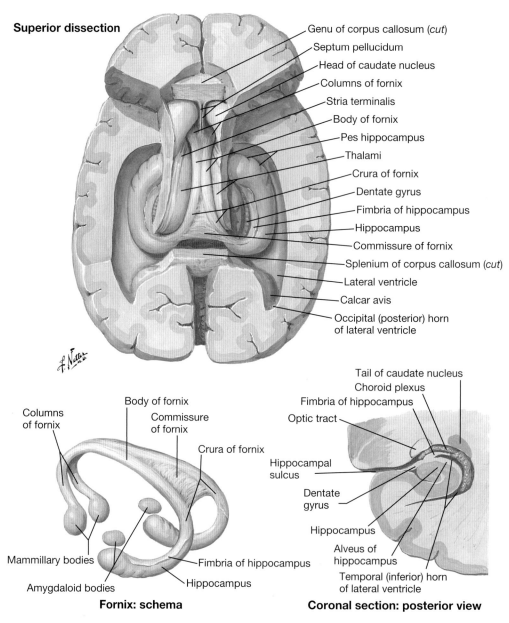

**Superior dissection**

Genu of corpus callosum (*cut*)
Septum pellucidum
Head of caudate nucleus
Columns of fornix
Stria terminalis
Body of fornix
Pes hippocampus
Thalami
Crura of fornix
Dentate gyrus
Fimbria of hippocampus
Hippocampus
Commissure of fornix
Splenium of corpus callosum (*cut*)
Lateral ventricle
Calcar avis
Occipital (posterior) horn of lateral ventricle

Columns of fornix
Body of fornix
Commissure of fornix
Crura of fornix
Mammillary bodies
Amygdaloid bodies
Fimbria of hippocampus
Hippocampus
**Fornix: schema**

Tail of caudate nucleus
Choroid plexus
Fimbria of hippocampus
Optic tract
Hippocampal sulcus
Dentate gyrus
Hippocampus
Alveus of hippocampus
Temporal (inferior) horn of lateral ventricle
**Coronal section: posterior view**

Figure 1.39 Hippocampus and fornix.
(Netter illustration from www.netterimages.com ©Elsevier Inc. All rights reserved.)

http://evolve.elsevier.com/AU/Bright/positioning/

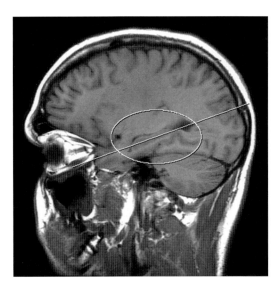

Figure 1.40 Location and alignment of the hippocampus in the temproal lobe.
(North Shore Radiology)

## Coils and patient considerations

Imaging of the temporal lobes is generally requested in cases of suspected hippocampal abnormality, evidenced by seizures and/or EEG anomalies. The hippocampus (circled in Figure 1.40, long axis indicated by the line) forms part of the limbic system along with the amygdala and olfactory cortex in the temporal lobe, as well as the hypothalamus and basal ganglia. The densely packed neurons of the hippocampus are subject to congenital malformation as well as damage due to mass lesions, diseases such as Alzheimer's and atrophy after infection or ischaemia; the result is memory impairment and/or seizure disorder.

Coronal images are the most important in the investigation of patients with epileptic disorders. Axial oblique images oriented to the temporal lobes are also useful, as well as imaging of the entire brain to rule out more systemic disease. The same imaging coil and patient considerations described in Chapter 1.1 should be applied.

# Imaging planes: Routine sequences

## Position:

- Supine, head first.

## Other considerations:

- The patient should be well padded to prevent image degradation or malalignment due to head movement.
- If the imaging coil has a mirror, ensure the patient is able to see out of the bore to alleviate claustrophobia.

## Coronal

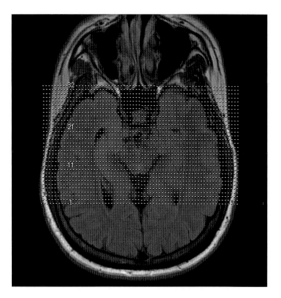

Figure 1.42 Coronal oblique planning on an axial image planned as described for temporal lobes on the next page.
(North Shore Radiology)

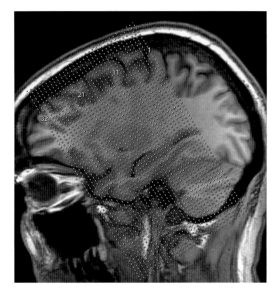

Figure 1.41 Coronal oblique planning on a sagittal image.
(North Shore Radiology)

## Alignment:

- Perpendicular to the hippocampus.

## Coverage:

*Superior to inferior:*
- Brainstem to vertex

*Lateral to medial:*
- Temporal bones on both sides

*Posterior to anterior:*
- Splenium of the corpus callosum to anterior temporal lobe.

## Demonstrates:

- Hippocampal morphology in short axis
- Relative atrophy or increase in size due to a mass lesion.

# Axial

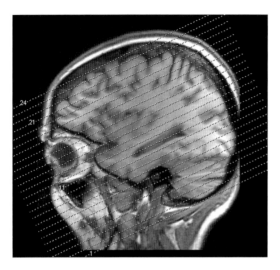

Figure 1.43 Axial oblique planning on a parasagittal image through the hippocampus.
(North Shore Radiology)

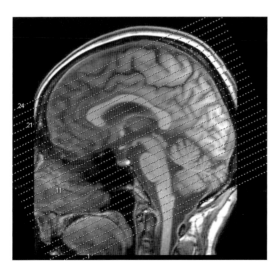

Figure 1.44 Axial oblique planning on a midsagittal image through the hippocampus.
(North Shore Radiology)

## Alignment:

- Parallel to the long axis of the hippocampus.
- This angle is much steeper than that prescribed for most routine brain scans and needs to be planned off a scan through the temporal lobes.

## Coverage:

*Superior to inferior:*
- Foramen magnum to vertex

*Lateral to medial:*
- Temporal bones on both sides

*Posterior to anterior:*
- Occipital to frontal lobes.

## Demonstrates:

- Hippocampal morphology in long axis.

# Chapter 1.8 Nasopharynx and sinuses

## Indications:

- Differentiation of benign lesions from malignant: this may include rhabdomyoma, papilloma, osteoma, neuroma, lipoma, fibroma, myxoma, neurofibromas, dermoid or Tornwaldt cyst
- Nasopharyngeal (NPC) or paranasal carcinoma, mostly in adults, e.g. squamous cell carcinoma (SCC), adenocarcinoma, lymphoma or sarcoma
- Metastases
- Glomus jugulare
- Inflammatory sinus disease/sinusitis +/− abscess or osteomyelitis.

## Coils and patient considerations

The frontal, maxillary, ethmoid and sphenoid sinuses are subject to numerous disease processes, with a tendency to progress within the interconnecting airways. Paediatric disease is most commonly benign in origin. Nasopharyngeal carcinoma, in particular, is an insidious disease most commonly affecting adult males of south-east Asian or North African heritage, although some children may also be affected. Patients generally have extension to the lymph nodes by the time of diagnosis and may also have associated invasion of the skull base, inducing cranial nerve disorders. Metastatic extension below the skull base may involve branches of cranial nerves $V_2$, $V_3$, VII, IX, X and XI. The full delineation of disease extent is crucial in determining the potential success of surgery; involvement of the prevertebral space often renders a lesion inoperable. Examination of the posterior fossa may also be required (see Ch 1.5).

A dedicated head coil should provide excellent coverage of the sinuses, skull base, oro- and nasopharynx. However if extension below the level of the mandibular ramus is suspected, a combined head and neck coil may be more appropriate (Fig I.6).

While local invasion of the sinuses, meninges, brain and soft tissues of the neck is common with carcinomas, benign lesions may also induce local damage through erosion of the bony surfaces. Care must be taken to ensure the full extent of disease is demonstrated in all planes. Computed tomography provides the best demonstration of sinus disease with disruption of the cortical bone, but MRI provides exquisite soft tissue detail that is often crucial in the management of more extensive and destructive disease of the nasopharynx more posteriorly.

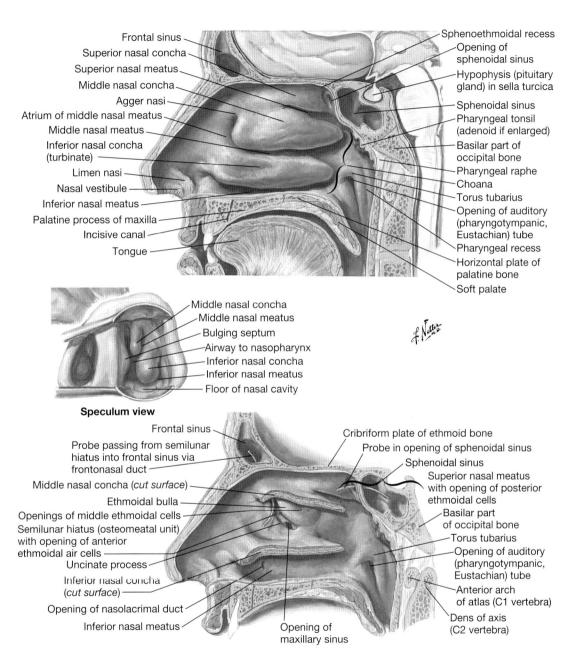

Frontal sinus
Superior nasal concha
Superior nasal meatus
Middle nasal concha
Agger nasi
Atrium of middle nasal meatus
Middle nasal meatus
Inferior nasal concha
(turbinate)
Limen nasi
Nasal vestibule
Inferior nasal meatus
Palatine process of maxilla
Incisive canal
Tongue

Sphenoethmoidal recess
Opening of
sphenoidal sinus
Hypophysis (pituitary
gland) in sella turcica
Sphenoidal sinus
Pharyngeal tonsil
(adenoid if enlarged)
Basilar part of
occipital bone
Pharyngeal raphe
Choana
Torus tubarius
Opening of auditory
(pharyngotympanic,
Eustachian) tube
Pharyngeal recess
Horizontal plate of
palatine bone
Soft palate

Middle nasal concha
Middle nasal meatus
Bulging septum
Airway to nasopharynx
Inferior nasal concha
Inferior nasal meatus
Floor of nasal cavity

**Speculum view**

Frontal sinus
Probe passing from semilunar
hiatus into frontal sinus via
frontonasal duct
Middle nasal concha (*cut surface*)
Ethmoidal bulla
Openings of middle ethmoidal cells
Semilunar hiatus (osteomeatal unit)
with opening of anterior
ethmoidal air cells
Uncinate process
Inferior nasal concha
(*cut surface*)
Opening of nasolacrimal duct
Inferior nasal meatus

Cribriform plate of ethmoid bone
Probe in opening of sphenoidal sinus
Sphenoidal sinus
Superior nasal meatus
with opening of posterior
ethmoidal cells
Basilar part
of occipital bone
Torus tubarius
Opening of auditory
(pharyngotympanic,
Eustachian) tube
Anterior arch
of atlas (C1 vertebra)
Dens of axis
(C2 vertebra)

Opening of
maxillary sinus

Figure 1.45 Mid sagittal section through the nasopharynx.
(Netter illustration from www.netterimages.com ©Elsevier Inc. All rights reserved.)

# Imaging planes: Routine sequences

## Position:

- Supine, head first.

## Other considerations:

- Patients may suffer nasal or sinus congestion, making breathing through the nose difficult. Suggest the patient keeps the mouth open to assist if this is easier during scanning.
- Between scans, offer the opportunity to swallow or clear the throat before continuing.

## Axial

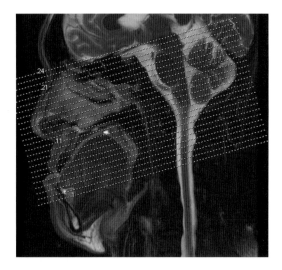

Figure 1.46  Axial planning on a sagittal image. (North Shore Radiology)

## Alignment:

- Parallel to the hard palate or airway. Check with your particular site.

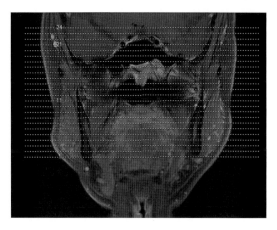

Figure 1.47  Axial planning on a coronal image. (North Shore Radiology)

## Coverage:

*Superior to inferior:*
- Nasopharynx: Mid cervical spine to cribriform plate (Figs 1.46 & 1.47)
- Sinuses: Floor of maxillary sinuses to superior aspect of the frontal sinus

*Lateral to medial:*
- Left to right mandibular rami

*Posterior to anterior:*
- Mid cervical spine to frontal and maxillary sinuses.

## Demonstrates:

- Disease extent and invasion of adjacent osseous boundaries
- Lymph node extension
- Integrity of the orbits
- Fluid levels within the sinuses.

# Coronal

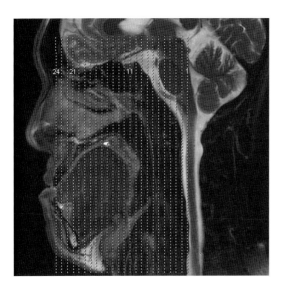

Figure 1.48 Coronal planning on a sagittal image. (North Shore Radiology)

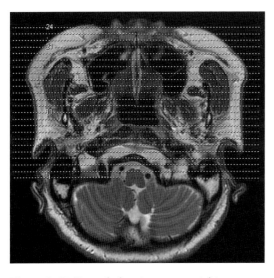

Figure 1.49 Coronal planning on an axial image. (North Shore Radiology)

## Alignment:

- Perpendicular to the hard palate.

## Coverage:

*Superior to inferior:*
- Nasopharynx: Parallel to posterior airway
- Sinuses: Floor of maxillary sinuses to superior aspect of the frontal sinus

*Lateral to medial:*
- Complete from left to right mandibular rami

*Posterior to anterior:*
- Mid cervical spine to frontal and maxillary sinuses.

## Demonstrates:

- Lateral spread
- Integrity of orbits
- Breach of integrity of osseous boundaries at the base of skull, including spread to cavernous sinuses
- Encroachment upon cranial nerves
- Malignant infiltration of lymph nodes.

# Imaging planes: Supplementary sequences

## Sagittal

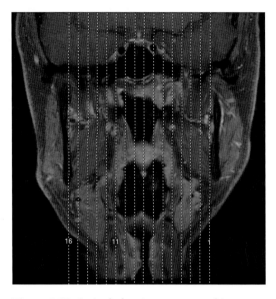

Figure 1.50 Sagittal planning on a coronal image.
(North Shore Radiology)

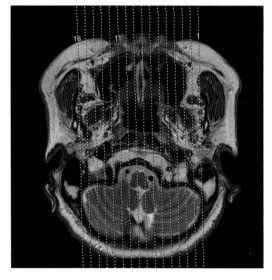

Figure 1.51 Sagittal planning on an axial image.
(North Shore Radiology)

## Alignment:

· True sagittal plane.

## Coverage:

· As per axial plane.

## Demonstrates:

· Best plane to demonstrate disruption of the cribriform plate
· Fluid levels within the sinuses
· Invasion of the clivus or pharyngobasilar fascia.

# Chapter 1.9 Temporomandibular joints

## Indications:

- Painful and/or clicking jaw
- Disc displacement or internal derangement
- Arthritis (most commonly RA, but also OA and infective)
- Post trauma
- Dislocation
- Congenital joint anomalies, such as condylar hypoplasia or agenesis
- Any of the diseases affecting synovial joints.

## Coils and patient considerations

The synovial joint between the mandibular condyle and the glenoid fossa of the temporal bone forms the temporomandibular joint (TMJ). A biconcave, cartilaginous meniscus or disc interposes the normally non-communicating superior and inferior compartments of this hinge joint. The superior and inferior lateral pterygoid muscles (LPM), extending from the inferior aspect of the greater sphenoid wing inferolaterally and posteroinferiorly, have variable attachments to the meniscus, mandibular condyle and pterygoid fovea, with a complex function that remains ill defined.

Damage to the supporting structures attached to this disc result in its displacement leading to joint dysfunction, women being more susceptible. Either hypertrophy or atrophy with contracture of the LPM may be associated with TMJ dysfunction. Disease is often bilateral, although the contralateral side may be asymptomatic; hence both sides should be examined simultaneously.

Investigation using a head coil may achieve acceptable results, but high quality scans of small joints such as these generally benefit from using an imaging coil of similarly small dimensions. A pair of coupled surface coils (Fig I.13) offer high spatial resolution and dedicated, simultaneous imaging of each joint.

Metallic dental implants should be removed prior to imaging when possible to assist in optimising field homogeneity.

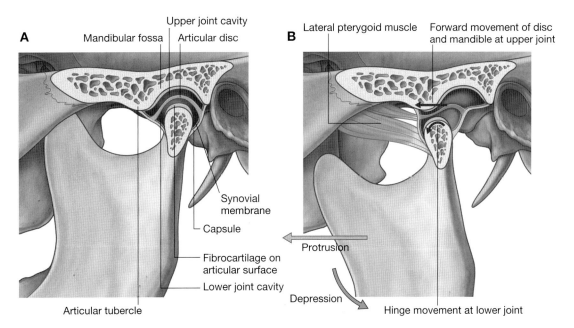

**Figure 1.52** The temporomandibular joint.
(From Drake, Gray's Anatomy for Students 2e, with permission)

# Imaging planes: Routine sequences

## Position:

- Supine, head first.

## Other considerations:

- Allow the patient the opportunity to swallow between imaging sequences, to prevent tongue and/or jaw motion degrading image quality.

## Sagittal or sagittal oblique

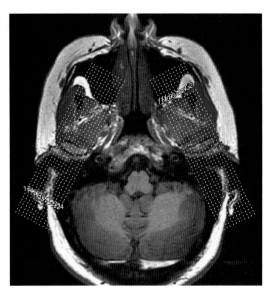

Figure 1.53 Biplane sagittal oblique planning on an axial image.
(North Shore Radiology)

## Alignment:

- Sagittal oblique (preferred orientation):
  - Perpendicular to the long axis of the mandibular condyle (Fig 1.53).
- Sagittal:
  - A true parasagittal plane.
- Scans usually performed with both closed and open mouth.

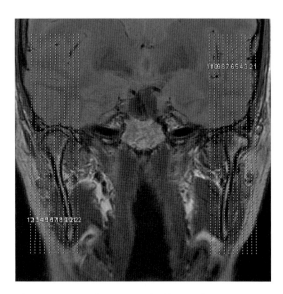

Figure 1.54 Biplane sagittal oblique planning on a coronal image.
(North Shore Radiology)

- For static open mouth scans, place a bite block between the teeth, asking the patient to hold it gently to assist in keeping the jaw still.
- Kinematic imaging may be performed, opening the mouth by incremental steps for each data set.

## Coverage:

*Superior to inferior:*
- Glenoid fossa to proximal mandibular ramus

*Lateral to medial:*
- Full width of the synovial joint
- The condyles move slightly lateral when the mouth opens; allow sufficient coverage to accommodate this translation

*Posterior to anterior:*
- Posterior aspect of the glenoid fossa to the articular eminence of the zygomatic eminence on each side.

# Demonstrates:

- Condylar and glenoid contour.
- Position and integrity of the meniscus, demonstrating the posterior and anterior bands of the disk, connected by the thinner intermediate or central zone.
- Sagittal:
  - May demonstrate fewer artefacts from permanent dental hardware than an oblique orientation.
- Kinematic scans demonstrate functional anatomy and disc displacement. Images may be viewed independently or as a cine loop.

# Coronal or coronal oblique

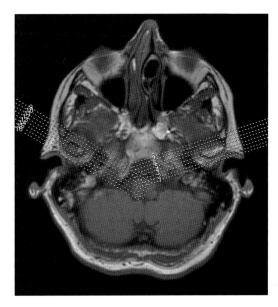

Figure 1.56 Coronal oblique planning on an axial image.
(North Shore Radiology)

## Alignment:

- Coronal:
  - Parallel to a line bisecting both condyles.
- Coronal oblique:
  - Parallel to the long axis of the mandibular condyle on an axial localiser
  - Mouth closed.

## Coverage:

- As for the sagittal oblique.

## Demonstrates:

- Condylar and glenoid contour
- Coronal oblique:
  - Best demonstrates medial or lateral disc displacement.

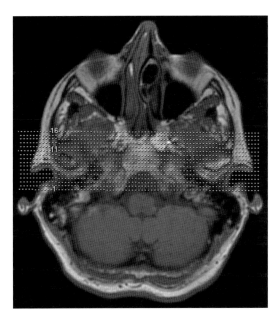

Figure 1.55 Coronal planning on an axial image.
(North Shore Radiology)

# Imaging planes: Supplementary sequences

## Sagittal oblique (condyle lateral-pterygoid muscle, CLPM)

### Alignment:

- Parallel to the long axis of the lateral pterygoid muscle, passing through the mandibular condyle
- Mouth closed.

### Coverage:

- As per routine sagittal oblique.

### Demonstrates:

- Anomalies of the lateral pterygoid muscle, which may account for TMJ dysfunction with or without demonstrated articular or meniscal disease.

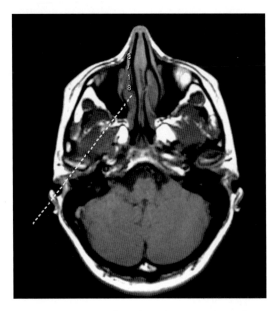

**Figure 1.57** Plane of the lateral pterygoid muscle. (North Shore Radiology)

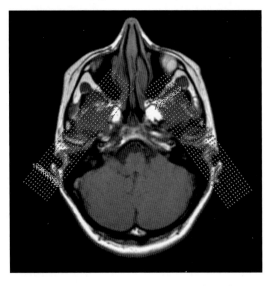

**Figure 1.58** Sagittal oblique planning, aligned to the lateral pterygoid muscle. (North Shore Radiology)

# Chapter 1.10 Soft tissue neck

## Indications:

- Carcinoma of the larynx and hypopharynx
- Benign lesions of the larynx
- Second or third branchial cleft cyst.

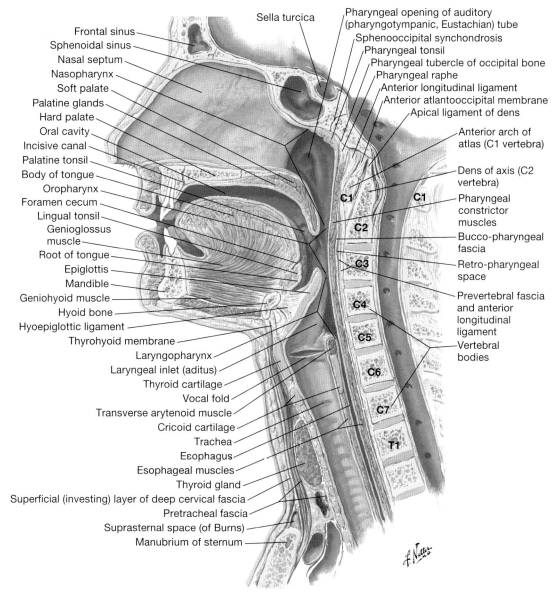

**Figure 1.59** Pharynx: median section.

(Netter illustration from www.netterimages.com ©Elsevier Inc. All rights reserved.)

http://evolve.elsevier.com/AU/Bright/positioning/

# Coils and patient considerations

Computed tomography is the preferred modality for imaging of this region, but MRI is useful in determining disease spread to the tongue and the cartilages of the throat. The radiofrequency coil of choice must provide good signal from the base of skull to the thoracic inlet (Figs I.5 & I.6).

Lesions in the airways of the neck are classified as supra- or subglottic. Depending on the point of origin within the larynx, malignancies may spread superiorly to the base of tongue, to the tissues anterior to the epiglottis including the laryngeal cartilages (hyoid, thyroid, corniculate, arytenoid and cricoid) and the true vocal cords inferiorly. Defining the extent of disease influences the choice of treatment method, as well as whether voice-sparing excision of a lesion (supraglottic) is possible versus complete laryngectomy.

The hypopharynx extends from the epiglottis (the inferior point of delineation for the oropharynx) to the cricoid cartilage. Disease of this tract is less common than in the respiratory tract, but carries a poor prognosis.

Metastatic nodal involvement is common in cancers of the head and neck. More than 300 nodes are found in this area, extending from the base of skull to thoracic inlet. Classification systems vary and are not discussed in this text, but the radiographer must be aware of the extent of possible disease spread to ensure comprehensive coverage.

# Imaging planes: Routine sequences

## Position:

- Supine, head first.

## Other considerations:

- Patients with diseases of the airways may suffer from respiratory discomfort that may be exacerbated in the supine position. Allowing the patient the opportunity to clear the throat between each pulse sequence may assist in generating images with limited motion artefact induced by swallowing or coughing.

## Axial

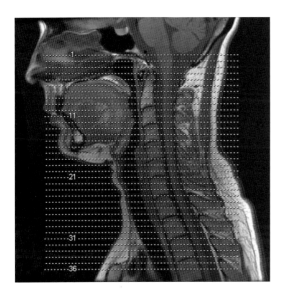

**Figure 1.60** Axial planning on a sagittal image. (North Shore Radiology)

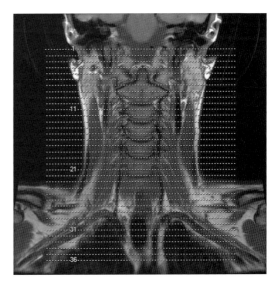

**Figure 1.61** Axial planning on a coronal image. (North Shore Radiology)

## Alignment:

- True axial plane.

## Coverage:

*Superior to inferior:*
- Base of skull to thoracic inlet

*Lateral to medial:*
- Mandibular rami on each side

*Posterior to anterior:*
- Skin surface of posterior neck and occiput to chin surface.

## Demonstrates:

- Sub mucosal spread between the hypopharynx and larynx
- Cartilage extension
- Encroachment upon and degree of encasement of the carotid artery by paraglottic tumour spread (may preclude surgical intervention).

# Coronal

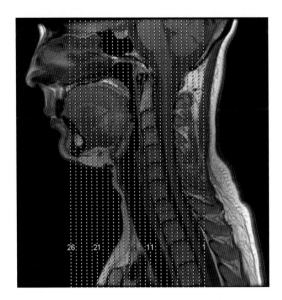

Figure 1.62 Coronal planning on a sagittal image.
(North Shore Radiology)

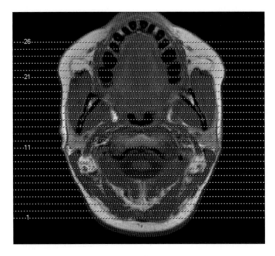

Figure 1.63 Coronal planning on an axial image.
(North Shore Radiology)

## Alignment:

· True coronal plane.

## Coverage:

· As for axial plane.

## Demonstrates:

· Disease extension lateral to the larynx
· Trans glottic spread (to involve the true vocal cords)
· Metastatic lymph nodes
· Disease extension to the neck cartilages or the false cords.

# Sagittal

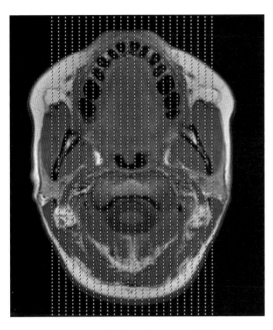

Figure 1.64 Sagittal planned on an axial image.
(North Shore Radiology)

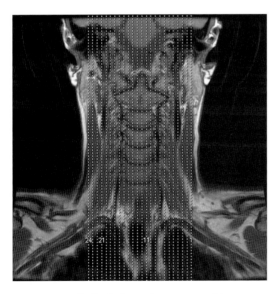

Figure 1.65 Sagittal planned on a coronal image.
(North Shore Radiology)

## Alignment:

- True sagittal plane.

## Coverage:

- As for axial plane.

## Demonstrates:

- Lesion spread to the base of tongue
- Disease extension to the neck cartilages or the false cords.

# Chapter 1.11 Brachial plexus

## Indications:

- Trauma
- Malignancy, e.g. primary nerve sheath tumour, metastatic deposits or direct invasion
- Benign tumour

- Neurofibromatosis
- Radiation fibrosis
- Thoracic outlet syndrome (also known as thoracic inlet syndrome).

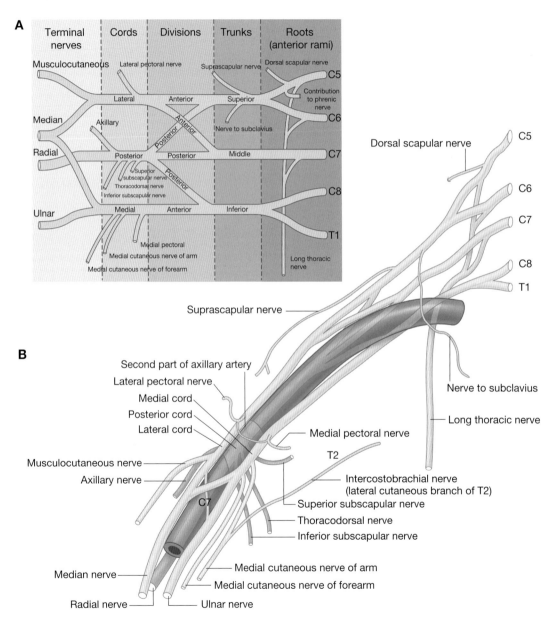

**Figure 1.66** The brachial plexus.
(From Drake, Gray's Anatomy for Students 2e, with permission)

# Coils and patient considerations

Spanning from the cervical spine to the gleno-humeral joint on both sides, imaging of the brachial plexus generally requires an imaging coil with a large field of view (Fig I.5). The complex anatomy of the brachial plexus begins with the exiting nerve roots of the lower cervical spine, with the roots of the fifth cervical to the first thoracic spinal nerves merging to form the upper, middle and lower trunks. The trunks divide to form anterior and posterior divisions that then merge to form the lateral, posterior and medial cords.

Two anomalous variations of nerve contribution may complicate imaging. The prefixed brachial plexus starts a level higher, involving the fourth to seventh cervical nerve roots. Conversely, a post-fixed plexus includes contributions from the sixth cervical nerve root to the second thoracic. To ensure complete imaging of the plexus, these potential anomalies should be borne in mind when planning scans.

Symptoms of brachial plexopathy can be difficult to distinguish from those of the cervical spine; it is not unusual for examination of both regions to be requested. In cases of traumatic nerve root avulsion, axial imaging of the cervical spine with a smaller field of view than for the brachial plexus is necessary to clearly demonstrate injury to the ventral and dorsal nerve roots within the spinal canal. Imaging of the cervical spine is discussed in Chapter 2.1.

# Imaging planes: Routine sequences

## Position:

- Supine, head first
- Arms by side
- Compression of neural or vascular structures may be best demonstrated by raising the arms above the head.

## Other considerations:

- The neurovascular coils can be quite intimidating to some patients. Most have a mirror that should be positioned so the patient can see out of the scanner bore.
- Make the patient as comfortable as possible, particularly if they have arm pain.

## Coronal

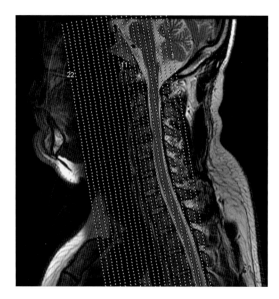

Figure 1.67 Coronal planning on a sagittal image. (North Shore Radiology)

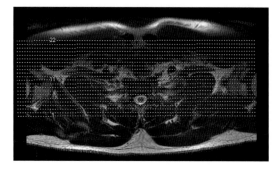

Figure 1.68 Coronal planning on an axial image. (North Shore Radiology)

## Alignment:

- True coronal plane.
- Angling the scans more anteriorly at the superior end may be preferred to try to capture the plexus in plane at the spine, as demonstrated above.
- This view may be repeated with the arms abducted and externally rotated (ABER) in cases of suspected thoracic outlet syndrome.

## Coverage:

*Superior to inferior:*
- Base of skull to fourth thoracic vertebra

*Lateral to medial:*
- Glenoid fossa on each side

*Posterior to anterior:*
- Spinous processes of the third cervical and second thoracic vertebrae through to the sternum.

## Demonstrates:

- In plane demonstration of both plexi
- Inflammation of the musculature
- Masses imposing upon or invading the plexus from the upper chest
- With arms raised, compression of neurovascular structures may be more clearly demonstrated.

## Axial

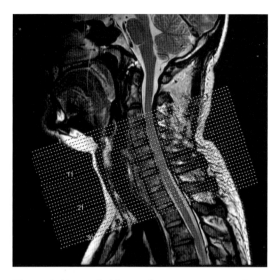

Figure 1.69 Axial oblique planning on a sagittal image.
(North Shore Radiology)

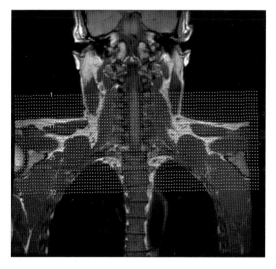

Figure 1.70 Axial oblique planning on a coronal image.
(North Shore Radiology)

## Alignment:

- Perpendicular to the long axis of the spinal cord.

## Coverage:

*Superior to inferior:*
- Third cervical to second thoracic vertebrae

*Lateral to medial:*
- Glenoid fossa on each side

*Posterior to anterior:*
- Spinous processes of the third cervical to the second thoracic vertebrae through to sternum.

## Demonstrates:

- Nerve roots exiting the spinal foramina and subsequent anatomy beyond (targeted, small field of view images should be performed for avulsion injuries).

# Sagittal

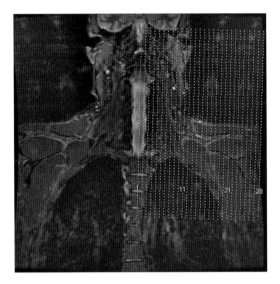

Figure 1.71 Sagittal planning on a coronal image. (North Shore Radiology)

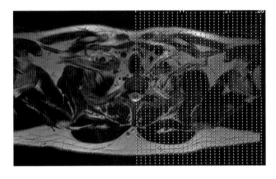

Figure 1.72 Sagittal planning on a sagittal image. (North Shore Radiology)

## Alignment:

- True sagittal plane
- This view may be repeated with the arms abducted and externally rotated in cases of suspected thoracic outlet syndrome.

## Coverage:

*Superior to inferior:*
- Base of skull to the fourth thoracic vertebrae

*Lateral to medial:*
- Mid-spinal cord to the glenoid fossa on each side

*Posterior to anterior:*
- Spinous processes of the third cervical to the second thoracic vertebrae through to sternum.

## Demonstrates:

- The neurovascular bundle in short axis, comprised of the trunks, division and cords of the plexus, in close association with the arteries supplying the upper limb.
- Arms raised, compression of neurovascular structures by anomalous anatomy may be apparent.

# Chapter 1.12 Head and neck vascular imaging

## Indications:

- Carotid, vertebral or cervical artery dissection or stenosis
- Horner's syndrome
- Known, suspected or family history of intracranial aneurysm
- Congenital vascular anomalies, e.g. Moyamoya disease or arteriovenous malformation (AVM)
- Thoracic outlet syndrome (also known as thoracic inlet syndrome)
- Trigeminal neuralgia.

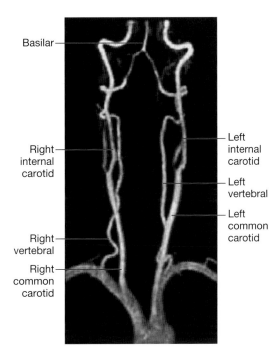

Figure 1.73 Arteries of the neck: maximum intensity projection.
(From Drake, Gray's Anatomy for Students 2e, with permission)

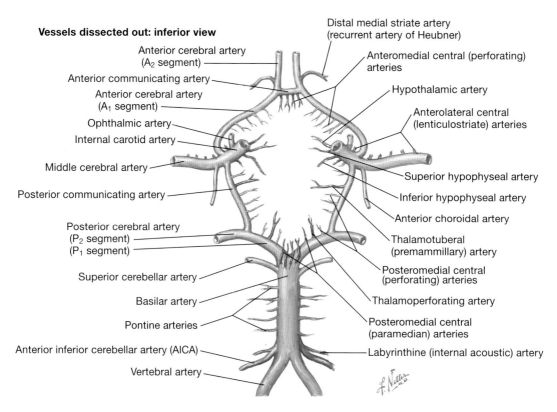

**Vessels dissected out: inferior view**

Distal medial striate artery
(recurrent artery of Heubner)

Anterior cerebral artery
($A_2$ segment)

Anterior communicating artery

Anterior cerebral artery
($A_1$ segment)

Ophthalmic artery

Internal carotid artery

Middle cerebral artery

Posterior communicating artery

Posterior cerebral artery
($P_2$ segment)
($P_1$ segment)

Superior cerebellar artery

Basilar artery

Pontine arteries

Anterior inferior cerebellar artery (AICA)

Vertebral artery

Anteromedial central (perforating)
arteries

Hypothalamic artery

Anterolateral central
(lenticulostriate) arteries

Superior hypophyseal artery

Inferior hypophyseal artery

Anterior choroidal artery

Thalamotuberal
(premammillary) artery

Posteromedial central
(perforating) arteries

Thalamoperforating artery

Posteromedial central
(paramedian) arteries

Labyrinthine (internal acoustic) artery

Figure 1.74 Arteries of the head.
(Netter illustration from www.netterimages.com ©Elsevier Inc. All rights reserved.)

## Coils and patient considerations

Magnetic resonance imaging of intracranial vascular pathology comes at a limited cost to time and equipment compared with interventional procedures. Modular coils extend the field of view to include imaging of vessels from the aortic arch to the circle of Willis (Fig I.5). Depending on the particular system in use, a dedicated head coil may be preferred.

Most frequently, the innominate artery branches off on the right side, from which the right common carotid and vertebral arteries arise. The left common carotid often originates directly from the aortic arch, with the left subclavian artery giving rise to the vertebral artery on that side.

The common carotid arteries divide into internal and external branches around the level of the angle of the mandible (third cervical vertebra). The internal carotid artery continues superiorly, entering the skull base via the carotid canal and progresses through the cavernous sinus. The artery divides into anterior, middle, posterior and choroidal arteries, the first three of which form the anterior portion of the circle of Willis.

The left and right vertebral arteries progress from the aortic arch and innominate arteries respectively, and enter the base of skull via the foramen magnum. Soon after they anastomose to form the short basilar artery behind the midbrain, before again dividing into the left and right posterior cerebral arteries. These two form the posterior circulation in the circle of Willis and often anastomose with the posterior communicating arteries.

The description of vascular supply to the neck and brain provided here is, at best, a template for the many variations that exist between individuals. In reality, vascular morphology is quite variable with the origins of the neck vessels and the completeness of the circle of Willis having been shown to be much less than uniform across the population. Identification of vascular origins, divisions and anastomoses is critical to patient management. As many vascular techniques result in the creation of maximum intensity projections (MIPs), the radiographer and reporting radiologist should be mindful of the potential loss of information from slow flow in the resultant composite images. This, in conjunction with the variable anatomical communications, should provide impetus to examine the raw data images for anomalous flow.

In-flow techniques without the use of intravenous (IV) contrast require imaging of vessels in the short axis. Conversely IV gadolinium allows imaging in-plane by exploiting shortened T1 times, making coronal imaging possible. Regardless of the imaging technique chosen, the coverage required remains unchanged.

# Imaging planes: Routine sequences

## Position:

- Supine, head first
- Arms by side.

## Other considerations:

- The neurovascular coils can be quite intimidating to some patients. Most have a mirror that should be positioned so that the patient can see out of the scanner bore.
- If scans involve two datasets for subtraction (e.g. mask and a contrast run), cannulate the patient before acquiring the mask. If the patient moves between the two datasets misregistration will detract from image quality.

## Axial: intracranial circulation

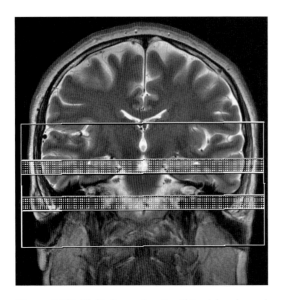

**Figure 1.75** Multiple overlapping thin slabs planned on a sagittal image.
(North Shore Radiology)

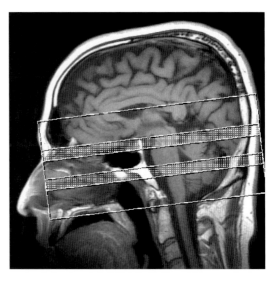

**Figure 1.76** Multiple overlapping thin slabs planned on a coronal image.
(North Shore Radiology)

## Alignment:

- Parallel to the cribriform plate
- Some sites may suggest angling the block so that the anterior portion is more superior to minimise susceptibility effects in the sphenoid sinus.

## Coverage:

*Superior to inferior:*
- Foramen magnum to genu of the corpus callosum

*Lateral to medial:*
- Full width of the hemispheres

*Posterior to anterior:*
- Occipital lobe to frontal lobe.

## Demonstrates:

- In-flow within the vertebrobasilar complex, circle of Willis, and out to the tertiary divisions of the internal carotid arteries.
- Volumes should be post processed to create MIPs.

# Axial: neck vessels

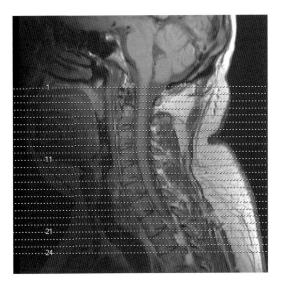

Figure 1.77 Axial planning on a sagittal image.
(North Shore Radiology)

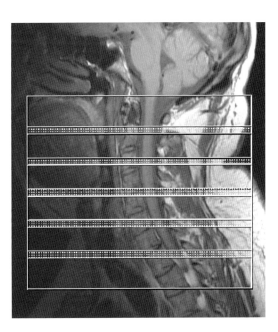

Figure 1.79 Multiple overlapping thin slabs planned on a sagittal image.
(North Shore Radiology)

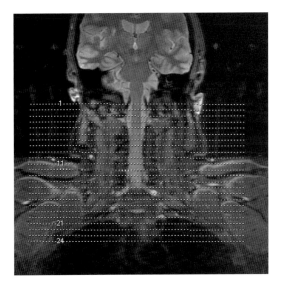

Figure 1.78 Axial planning on a coronal image.
(North Shore Radiology)

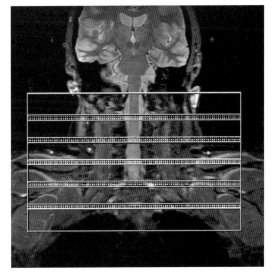

Figure 1.80 Multiple overlapping thin slabs planned on a coronal image.
(North Shore Radiology)

## Alignment:

- True axial plane.

## Coverage:

*Superior to inferior:*
- Aortic arch to base of skull

*Lateral to medial:*
- Mid clavicles on each side

*Posterior to anterior:*
- Occipital lobe to the anterior skin surface of neck.

## Demonstrates:

- Two-dimensional axial scans are preferred for demonstration of intramural thrombus or haematoma, particularly when using a T1 fat suppressed pulse sequence (Figs 1.77 & 1.78).
- Three-dimensional overlapping thin slab volumes should be post processed to create MIPs (Figs 1.79 & 1.80).

# Coronal: neck vessels

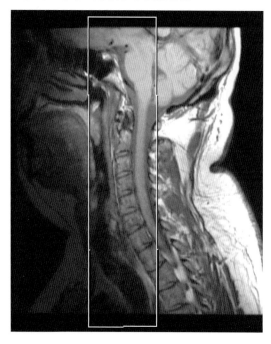

**Figure 1.81** Coronal volume planned on a sagittal image.
(North Shore Radiology)

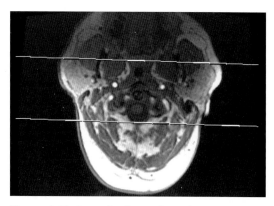

**Figure 1.82** Coronal volume planned on an axial image.
(North Shore Radiology)

## Alignment:

- Coronal to the long axis of the vessels of the neck.
- Scans may be obliqued, depending on the degree of tortuosity and curvature of the neck vessels.
- Planning may be better achieved by using a good quality axial 2D dataset, scrolling through the images to be sure the vessels are adequately covered along their entire length.
- This scan requires dynamic imaging with IV contrast.

## Coverage:

*Superior to inferior:*
- Aortic arch to base of skull

*Lateral to medial:*
- Proximal innominate artery to proximal left subclavian artery

*Posterior to anterior:*
- Posterior communicating artery to carotid siphons, including the aortic arch inferiorly.

## Demonstrates:

- Stenosis
- Dissection
- Data should be post processed as MIPs.

# Further reading

Adamczyk M, Bulski T, Sowinska J et al 2007 Trigeminal nerve–artery contact in people without trigeminal neuralgia: MR study. Medical Science Monitor 13(Supp1):38–43

Alford BR 2006 Department of Otolaryngology–Head and Neck Surgery, Core Curriculum Syllabus: Review of Anatomy—The Larynx, Baylor College of Medicine, 23 Jan. Online. Available: http://www.bcm.edu/oto/index.cfm?pmid=15473; 17 Mar 2011

Blair DN, Rapoport S, Sostman HD et al 1987 Normal brachial plexus: MR imaging. Radiology 167(3):763–767

Bumann A, Lotzmann U 2002 TMJ Disorders and Orofacial Pain: The Role of Dentistry in a Multidisciplinary Diagnostic Approach. Thieme, Stuttgart, pp.11, 141–160

Castagno AA, Shuman WP 1987 MR imaging in clinically suspected brachial plexus tumor. American Journal of Roentgenology 149(6):1219–1222

Castillo M 2005 Imaging the anatomy of the brachial plexus: Review and self-assessment module. American Journal of Roentgenology 85(6 Suppl):S196–204

Chong V 2004 Cervical lymphadenopathy: What radiologists need to know. Cancer Imaging 4:116–120

Collins JD, Disher AC, Miller TQ et al 1995 The anatomy of the brachial plexus as displayed by magnetic resonance imaging: technique and application. Journal of the National Medical Association 87(7):489–498

Comoretto M, Balestreri L, Borsatti E et al 2008 Detection and restaging of residual and/or recurrent nasopharyngeal carcinoma after chemotherapy and radiation therapy: Comparison of MR imaging and FDG PET/CT. Radiology 249(1):203–211

Connor S 2007 Laryngeal cancer: How does the radiologist help? Cancer Imaging 28(7):93–103

Cottier JP, Destrieux C, Brunereau L et al 2000 Cavernous sinus invasion by pituitary adenoma: MR imaging. Radiology 215:463–469

Demondion X, Boutry N, Drizenko A et al 2000 Thoracic outlet: Anatomic correlation with MR imaging. American Journal of Roentgenology 175(2):417–422

Demondion X, Herbinet P, Van Sint Jan S et al 2006 Imaging assessment of thoracic outlet syndrome. Radiographics 26(6):1735–1750

Gao FQ, Black SE, Leibovitch FS et al 2003 A reliable MR measurement of medial temporal lobe width from the Sunnybrook Dementia Study. Neurobiology and Aging 24(1):49–56

Gronseth G, Cruccu G, Alksne C et al 2008 Practice parameter: the diagnostic evaluation and treatment of trigeminal neuralgia (an evidence-based review): Report of the Quality Standards Subcommittee of the American Academy of Neurology and the European Federation of Neurological Societies. Neurology 71(15):1183–1190

Hetts SW, Sherr EH, Chao S et al 2006 Anomalies of the Corpus Callosum: An MR analysis of the phenotypic spectrum of associated malformations. American Journal of Roentgenology 187:1343–1348

Huff JS 2009 Trigeminal neuralgia. emedicine. Online. Available: http://emedicine.medscape.com/article/794402-print; 14 Mar 2011

Kamel HAM, Toland J 2001 Trigeminal nerve anatomy: Illustrated using examples of abnormalities. American Journal of Roentgenology 176:247–251

Kattah J, Pula J 2009 Cavernous sinus syndromes. emedicine. Online. Available: http://emedicine.

medscape.com/article/1161710-print; 14 Mar 2011

Khan AN, Haque SU, MacDonald S et al 2008 Temporomandibular joint, meniscus abnormalities. emedicine. Available http://emedicine.medscape.com/article/385129-overview; 14 Mar 2011

King AD, Lam WWM, Leung SF et al 1999 MRI of local disease in nasopharyngeal carcinoma: Tumour extent vs tumour stage. British Journal of Radiology 72:734–741

Ko DY, Sahai-Srivastava S 2009 Temporal lobe epilepsy. emedicine. Online. Available: http://emedicine.medscape.com/article/1184509-print; 14 Mar 2011

Krabbe-Hartkamp MJ, ven der Grond J, de Leeuw FE et al 1998 Circle of Willis: morphologic variation on three-dimensional time-of-flight MR angiograms. Radiology 207(1):103–110

Kutz JW, Roland PS, Isaacson B 2009 Skull Base, Acoustic neuroma (vestibular schwannoma). emedicine. Online. Available: http://emedicine.medscape.com/article/882876-print; 14 Mar 2011

Kwan TL, Tang KW, Pak KKT et al 2004 Screening for vestibular schwannoma by magnetic resonance imaging: Analysis of 1821 patients. Hong Kong Medical Journal 10(1):38–43

Layton KF, Kallmes DF, Cloft HJ et al 2006 Bovine aortic arch variant in humans: clarification of a common misnomer. American Journal of Neuroradiology 7:1541–1542

Lee SH, Rao, Krishna, KCVG, Zimmerman RA. 1999 Anatomy. In: Cranial MRI and CT. 4th edn McGraw-Hill, New York, 114–117

Mack MG, Vogl TJ 1999 MR imaging of the head and neck. European Radiology 9:1247–1251

Mathai KI, Sengupta SK et al 2009 Hearing preservation in a case of acoustic schwannoma. Medical Journal Armed Forces India 65:290–291

Naidich TP, Daniels DL, Haughton VM et al 1987 Hippocampal formation and related structures of the limbic lobe: Anatomic-MR correlation; Part I. Surface features and coronal sections. Radiology 162(3):747–754

Ng SH, Chang TC, Ko SF et al 1997 Nasopharyngeal carcinoma: MRI and CT assessment. Neuroradiology 39:741–746

Ono K, Arai H, Endo T et al 2004 Detailed anatomy of the abducent nerve: Evagination of CSF into Dorello canal. American Journal of Neuroradiology 25:623–626

Paulino AC, Grupp SA 2008 Nasopharyngeal cancer. emedicine. Online. Available: http://emedicine.medscape.com/article/988165-print; 14 Mar 2011

Pluta RM, Luliano BA 2009 Glomus tumours. emedicine. Online. Available: http://emedicine.medscape.com/article/251009-print; 14 Mar 2011

Posniak HV, Olson MC, Dudiak CM et al 1993 MR imaging of the brachial plexus. American Journal of Roentgenology 161(2):373–379

Rodallec MH, Marteau V, Gerber S et al 2008 Craniocervical arterial dissection: Spectrum of imaging findings and differential diagnosis. RadioGraphics 28(6):1711–1728

Roth C, Ward RJ, Tsai S et al 2005 MR imaging of the TMJ: A pictorial essay. Applied Radiology 34(5):9–16 [In Medscape Today, 25 Mar 2005]

Rubinstein D, Sandberg EJ, Cajade-Law AG 1996 Anatomy of the facial and vestibulocochlear nerves in the internal auditory canal. American Journal of Neuroradiology 17:1099–1105

Sadhev A, Reznek RH, Evanson J et al 2007 Imaging in Cushing's Syndrome. Arquivos Brasileiros de Endocrinologia e Metabologia 51(8):1319–1328

Saleem SN, Ahmed-Hesham MS, Lee DHL 2007 Lesions of the hypothalamus: MR imaging diagnostic features. Radiographics 27:1087–1108

Salzman KL, Davidson CH, Harnsberger HR et al 2001 Dumbbell schwannomas of the internal auditory canal. American Journal of Neuroradiology 22:1368–1376

Saxton EH, Theodore TQ, Collins JD 1999 Migraine complicated by brachial plexopathy as displayed by MRI and MRA: Aberrant subclavian artery and cervical ribs. Journal of the National Medical Association 91(6):333–341

Shellock FG 2003 Functional assessment of the joints using kinematic magnetic resonance imaging. Seminars in Musculoskeletal Radiology 7(4):249–276

Som PM, Curtin HD Various chapters. In: Head and Neck Imaging, Volume One. 4th ed. St. Louis: Mosby; 2003:124, 150–3, 995–1010

Stark DD, Bradley WG, 1999 Chapter 82. In: Magnetic Resonance Imaging, Volume III, 3rd ed. St. Louis: Mosby; 1785–1793

Stritch School of Medicine 2009 Structure of the Human body: Cranial Nerves Summary. Loyola University Medical Education Network Chicago. Online. Available: http://www.meddean.luc.edu/lumen/MedED/grossanatomy/h_n/cn/cn1/table1.htm; 14 Mar 2011

Tomas X, Pomes J, Berenguer J et al 2006 MR imaging of temporomandibular dysfunction: A pictorial review. Radiographics 26(3):765–781

Weedman Molavi, D 1997 Neuroscience Tutorial: Medial Temporal Lobe and Memory. Washington University School of Medicine. Online. Available: http://thalamus.wustl.edu/course/limbic.html; 14 Mar 2011

Weissman JL, Hirsch BE 2000 Imaging of tinnitus: A review. Radiology 216:342–349

Woolfall P, Coulthard A 2001 Trigeminal nerve: Anatomy and pathology. British Journal of Radiology 74:458–467

Wong W [no date] Deep Spaces, Paranasal sinuses and nasopharynx. Online. Available: http://spinwarp.ucsd.edu/neuroweb/Text/ent-230.htm; 14 Mar 2011

Yamada I, Matsushima Y, Suzuki S 1992 Moyamoya Disease: Diagnosis with three-dimensional time-of-flight MR angiography. Radiology 184(3):773–778

Yang X 2002 Magnetic resonance imaging of the lateral pterygoid muscle in temporomandibular disorders. Yliopisto: University of Oulu. Online. Available: http://herkules.oulu.fi/isbn9514266439/html/index.html; 14 Mar 2011

Yoshino N, Akimoto H, Yamada I et al 2003 Trigeminal Neuralgia: Evaluation of Neuralgic Manifestation and Site of Neurovascular Compression with 3D CISS MR imaging and MR angiography. Radiology 228:539–545

Yousem DM, Hatabu H, Hurst RW et al 1995 Carotid artery invasion by head and neck masses: Prediction with MR imaging. Radiology 195:715–720

Zink E 2005 Recognizing and intervening in pituitary apoplexy. Medscape Today. Online. Available: http://www.medscape.com/viewarticle/518323_3; 14 Mar 2011

# Section 2

# Spine

# Chapter 2.1 Cervical spine

## Indications:

- Radiculopathy
- Myelopathy
- Disc lesion
- Whiplash
- Arthritis (RA or OA)

- Syringomyelia/syrinx
- Primary malignancy, e.g. ependymoma
- Secondary malignancy, e.g. germinoma
- Benign tumour, e.g. meningioma
- Demyelination, e.g. MS.

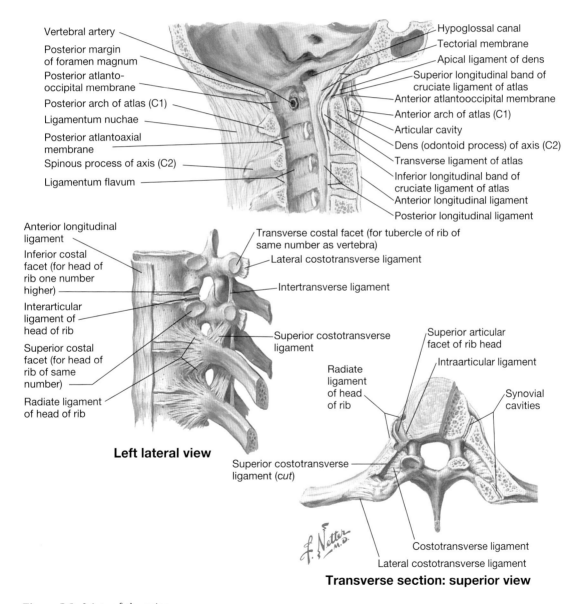

**Figure 2.1** Joints of the spine.

(Netter illustration from www.netterimages.com ©Elsevier Inc. All rights reserved.)

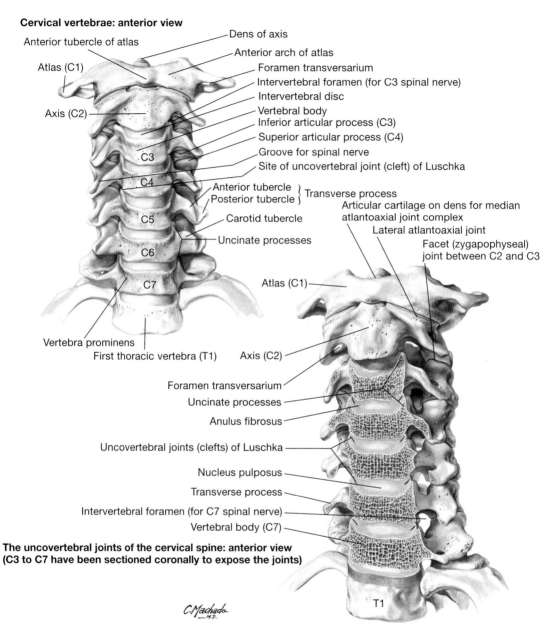

**Cervical vertebrae: anterior view**

- Anterior tubercle of atlas
- Atlas (C1)
- Axis (C2)
- C3
- C4
- C5
- C6
- C7
- Vertebra prominens
- First thoracic vertebra (T1)

- Dens of axis
- Anterior arch of atlas
- Foramen transversarium
- Intervertebral foramen (for C3 spinal nerve)
- Intervertebral disc
- Vertebral body
- Inferior articular process (C3)
- Superior articular process (C4)
- Groove for spinal nerve
- Site of uncovertebral joint (cleft) of Luschka
- Anterior tubercle } Transverse process
- Posterior tubercle }
- Carotid tubercle
- Uncinate processes

- Articular cartilage on dens for median atlantoaxial joint complex
- Lateral atlantoaxial joint
- Facet (zygapophyseal) joint between C2 and C3
- Atlas (C1)
- Axis (C2)
- Foramen transversarium
- Uncinate processes
- Anulus fibrosus
- Uncovertebral joints (clefts) of Luschka
- Nucleus pulposus
- Transverse process
- Intervertebral foramen (for C7 spinal nerve)
- Vertebral body (C7)
- T1

**The uncovertebral joints of the cervical spine: anterior view (C3 to C7 have been sectioned coronally to expose the joints)**

*C. Machado M.D.*

Figure 2.2 The cervical column.

(Netter illustration from www.netterimages.com ©Elsevier Inc. All rights reserved.)

## Coils and patient considerations

Exiting the cranium via the foramen magnum, the spinal cord is contained within the vertebral column. It gives off nerves on each side between each of the bones in the spine, commencing with the first cervical nerve root between the base of the skull and the first cervical vertebra. There are eight cervical nerves roots in all, the eighth exiting between the seventh and eighth cervical vertebrae.

Intervertebral discs between each vertebra, commencing at the C2/3 level, facilitate flexibility of movement, cushion the bones from shock, and assist in maintaining alignment.

Ligaments supporting the spine include the anterior and posterior longitudinal, intimately attached to the bodies of the vertebrae. The former commences at the base of the skull and extends the full length of the vertebral column to the sacrum. The posterior ligament is within the spinal canal, running along the posterior aspect of the vertebral bodies from the second cervical vertebra to the sacrum.

Connecting the laminae of each of the vertebral bodies from C2 to S1 are the ligamentum flava. The intertransverse and interspinous ligaments connect the transverse processes and spinous processes of the vertebrae, respectively. Finally, the nuchal ligament extends from the occiput to the spinous process of the seventh cervical vertebra. The vertebral arteries course through the transverse foramen of the sixth to first cervical vertebra.

Imaging coils often facilitate imaging of the head as well as the neck, with modular elements that may be attached as required (Figs I.4, I.5 & I.6).

For many, lying supine can exacerbate their pain, particularly if they are kyphotic. Placing a pillow or two beneath the patient's buttocks allows the upper thoracic spine and neck to lie more horizontally for imaging of the superior part of the spine. A large bolster under the knees supports the lower half of the body, while a small sponge beneath the head can alleviate neck strain.

# Imaging planes: Routine sequences

## Position:

- Supine, head first.

## Other considerations:

- The head should be immobilised with padding in a neutral position, not rotated to one side.

## Sagittal

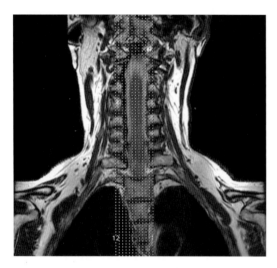

**Figure 2.3** Sagittal planned on a coronal image.
(North Shore Radiology)

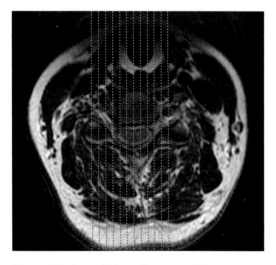

**Figure 2.4** Sagittal planned on an axial image.
(North Shore Radiology)

## Alignment:

- Parallel to the long axis of the spinal cord.
- This plane is generally performed in a neutral position, however rapid scans in flexion and extension may also be required. Use sponges to support and stabilise the head and neck in each position.

## Coverage:

*Superior to inferior:*
- Craniocervical junction to second thoracic vertebra

*Lateral to medial:*
- Vertebral pedicles on each side

*Posterior to anterior:*
- Spinous processes to prevertebral tissues.

## Demonstrates:

- Vertebral alignment
- Bony integrity and end plate disruption
- Herniated disc +/− impingement on nerve roots
- Space occupying lesions within the spinal canal, canal stenosis
- Ligamentum flavum
- Syrinx
- Subluxation caused by erosion and pannus formation of the dens due to RA
- Flexion-extension:
  - instability at the craniocervical junction in RA
  - cord impingement induced or worsened by position, particularly in extension.

# Axial

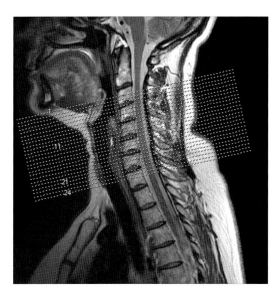

Figure 2.5 Axial planned on a sagittal image.
(North Shore Radiology)

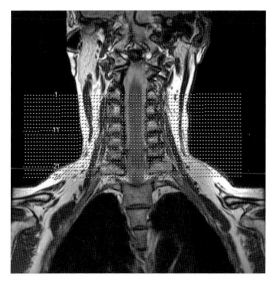

Figure 2.6 Axial planned on a coronal image.
(North Shore Radiology)

## Alignment:

- Perpendicular to the long axis of the cervical cord.

## Coverage:

*Superior to inferior:*
- Pedicle of the third cervical vertebra to the pedicle of the first thoracic vertebra
- Post trauma, scans should commence at the base of the skull

*Lateral to medial:*
- Intervertebral foramina on each side

*Posterior to anterior:*
- Spinous processes to prevertebral tissues.

## Demonstrates:

- Herniated disc +/− impingement on nerve roots
- Space occupying lesions within the spinal canal
- Syrinx
- Paravertebral extension of masses into the soft tissues.

# Imaging planes: Supplementary sequences

## Coronal

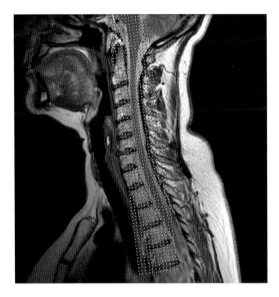

**Figure 2.7** Coronal planned on a sagittal iimage.
(North Shore Radiology)

## Alignment:

- Parallel to the long axis of the spinal cord. Some obliquity will most likely be required to achieve this.

## Coverage:

*Superior to inferior:*
- Craniocervical junction to the second thoracic vertebra

*Lateral to medial:*
- Transverse processes on each side

*Posterior to anterior:*
- Entire vertebral foramen to midway through the vertebral bodies.

## Demonstrates:

- Torticollis or scoliosis
- Space occupying lesions within the spinal canal
- Syrinx
- Lateral compression of nerve roots.

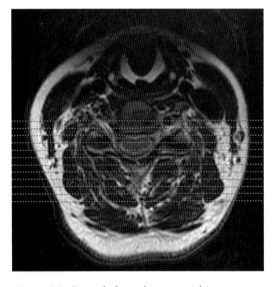

**Figure 2.8** Coronal planned on an axial image.
(North Shore Radiology)

# Sagittal oblique

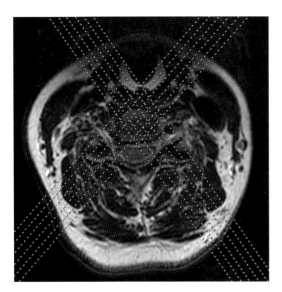

Figure 2.9 Sagittal oblique planned on an axial image.
(North Shore Radiology)

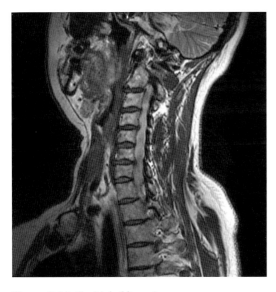

Figure 2.10 Sagittal oblique image.
(North Shore Radiology)

## Alignment:

- Perpendicular to the nerve roots as they exit the cervical canal in the mid cervical spine. An angle of approximately 45° should be expected.
- Verify that the slices will cover the nerve roots and foramina on each side at the superior and inferior cervical spine.
- Bilateral scans may be performed simultaneously or separately.

## Coverage:

*Superior to inferior:*
- Craniocervical junction to the first thoracic vertebra

*Lateral to medial:*
- Nerve root origins at the edge of the cervical cord to the lateral aspect of the spinal foramen

*Posterior to anterior:*
- Entire vertebral foramen to midway through the vertebral bodies.

## Demonstrates:

- Impingement of disc lesion on nerve roots, shown en face, as they exit via the spinal foramina
- Complementary to the axial images, this view assists in demonstrating the severity of foraminal impingement.

# Chapter 2.2 Thoracic spine

## Indications:

- Myelopathy
- Radiculopathy
- Herniated disc
- Syringomyelia/syrinx
- Primary malignancy, e.g. ependymoma
- Secondary malignancy, e.g. germinoma, drop metastases
- Benign tumour, e.g. meningioma
- Demyelination, e.g. MS
- Scoliosis.

## Coils and patient considerations

Extending from the seventh cervical vertebra, the supraspinal ligament continues in place of the nuchal ligament of the cervical spine. It terminates at the scarum. The remaining ligaments are similar to those described in Chapter 2.1. There are twelve paired thoracic nerve roots exiting the spinal column.

Imaging of the thoracic spine is often performed in conjunction with the cervical spine, but where a discrete solitary lesion is the source of pathology, limited scans of this region may be requested. At least one sagittal scan that overlaps with a scan of the cervical spine should be performed to determine vertebral levels. Alternately, one pulse sequence that covers from the craniocervical junction to the first lumbar vertebra may be performed. A marker placed on the skin within the field of view or a digital measurement demonstrating overlap between the fields of view should be used to verify that complete coverage has been achieved (Figs 2.12 & 2.13). Most spine coils will accommodate imaging of all regions from occiput to coccyx (Fig I.4).

Tilting the patient back to accommodate kyphosis as described in Chapter 2.1 can limit signal in the thoracic region, as the spine may be too distant from the surface detectors. It may be necessary to compromise, tilting back a little and supporting the head.

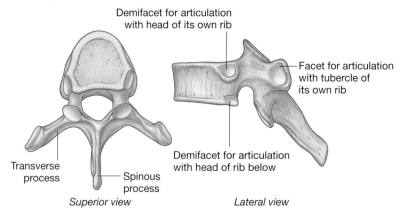

Demifacet for articulation
with head of its own rib

Facet for articulation
with tubercle of
its own rib

Transverse
process

Spinous
process

Demifacet for articulation
with head of rib below

*Superior view*                    *Lateral view*

Figure 2.11 A portion of the thoracic vertebral column.
(from Drake, Gray's Anatomy for Students 2e, with permission)

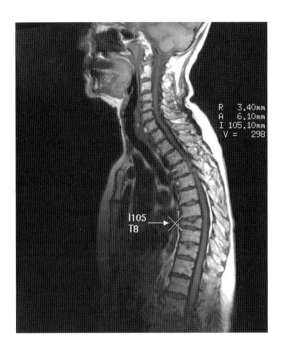

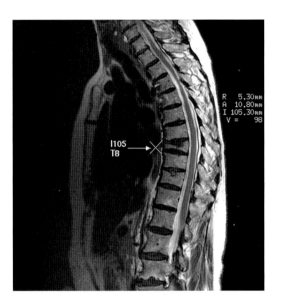

Figure 2.13 Establishing a vertebral level using a digital marker by comparing against Figure 2.12.
(North Shore Radiology)

Figure 2.12 Marking a vertebral level on an image from which C1 can be established. This can be used for comparison.
(North Shore Radiology)

# Imaging planes: Routine sequences

## Position:

- Supine, head first.

## Other considerations:

- The head should be immobilised with padding in a neutral position, not rotated to one side.

## Sagittal

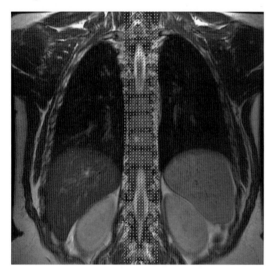

**Figure 2.14** Sagittal planned on a coronal image. (North Shore Radiology)

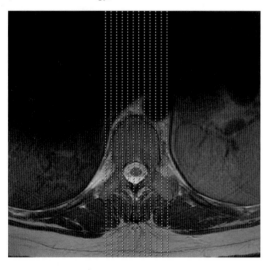

**Figure 2.15** Sagittal planned on an axial image. (North Shore Radiology)

## Alignment:

- Parallel to the long axis of the spinal cord.

## Coverage:

*Superior to inferior:*
- Seventh cervical vertebra to first lumbar vertebra
- If the conus is not fully demonstrated, sagittal scans should be done of the lumbar spine to ensure that a tethered cord is not missed

*Lateral to medial:*
- Vertebral pedicles on each side

*Posterior to anterior:*
- Spinous processes to prevertebral tissues.

## Demonstrates:

- Vertebral alignment, bony integrity and encroachment of retropulsed fragments on the spinal canal
- Cord displacement within the canal due to cord herniation or an intradural mass
- End plate disruption
- Syrinx
- Herniated disc
- Space occupying lesions within the spinal canal
- Ligamentum flava hypertrophy
- Conus.

# Axial

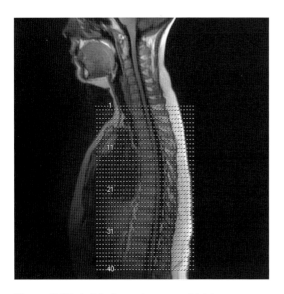

Figure 2.16 Axial planned on a sagittal image demonstrating C1, ensuring complete coverage of the thoracic cord.
(North Shore Radiology)

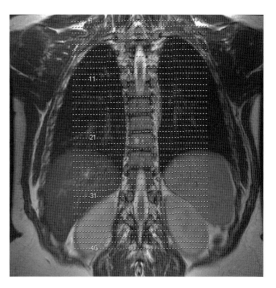

Figure 2.18 Axial planned on a coronal image.
(North Shore Radiology)

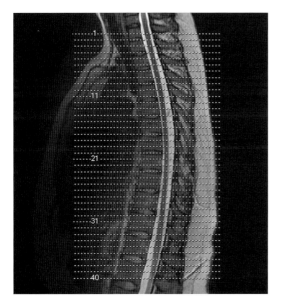

Figure 2.17 Axial planned on a sagittal image.
(North Shore Radiology)

## Alignment:

- Perpendicular to the long axis of the thoracic cord
- Where significant kyphosis is apparent, two groups planned at differing angles perpendicular to the spine may be preferred.

## Coverage:

*Superior to inferior:*
- As required by the radiologist, covering from the pedicles of one vertebra above and below the vertebrae of interest, e.g if T8–10 are of interest, scan from the pedicles of T7 to T11.
- If there is not a specific level to investigate, wider spaced axial scans throughout the thoracic spine may be acceptable.

*Lateral to medial:*
- Intervertebral foramina on each side

*Posterior to anterior:*
- Spinous processes to prevertebral tissues.

## Demonstrates:

- Herniated disc
- Canal stenosis
- Space occupying lesions within the spinal canal
- Paravertebral extension of masses into the soft tissues
- Syrinx.

# Imaging planes: Supplementary sequences

## Coronal

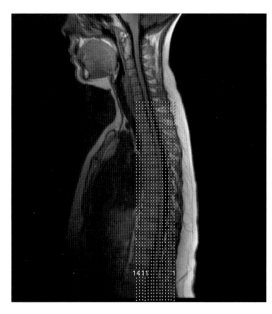

Figure 2.19 Coronal planned on a sagittal image.
(North Shore Radiology)

## Alignment:

- Parallel to the long axis of the spinal cord. Some obliquity will most likely be required to achieve this.

## Coverage:

*Superior to inferior:*
- Seventh cervical vertebra to the first lumbar vertebra

*Lateral to medial:*
- Transverse processes on each side

*Posterior to anterior:*
- Entire vertebral foramen to midway through the vertebral bodies of C7 and L1.

## Demonstrates:

- Scoliosis
- Space-occupying lesions within the spinal canal
- Syrinx
- Compression laterally on the nerve roots.

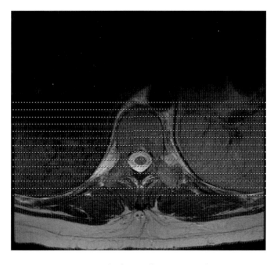

Figure 2.20 Coronal planned on an axial image.
(North Shore Radiology)

# Chapter 2.3 Lumbar spine

## Indications:

- Radiculopathy
- Sciatica
- Myelopathy
- Herniated disc
- Arthritis (RA or OA)
- Tethered cord
- Primary malignancy, e.g. ependymoma
- Secondary malignancy, e.g. germinoma
- Benign tumour, e.g. meningioma
- Cauda equina syndrome.

## Coils and patient considerations

The ligaments of the lumbar region have been described in Chapters 2.1 and 2.2. The spinal cord terminates between the eleventh thoracic and first lumbar vertebrae, at which point the cauda equina forms. The cauda equina produces the five lumbar nerves and continues into the scarum. A spine coil will provide coverage from occiput to coccyx (Fig I.4).

Kyphotic patients may need extra support under the head and upper spine, and many appreciate a sponge beneath the knees. Extending the legs may exacerbate pain due to a disc lesion compressing a nerve root.

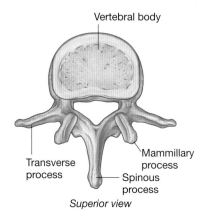

*Superior view*

Figure 2.21  Ligaments of the lumbar spine.
(from Drake, Gray's Anatomy for Students 2e, with permission)

# Imaging planes: Routine sequences

## Position:

- Supine, head or feet first.

## Other considerations:

- Support the head with a pillow or sponges.
- A feet-first orientation may be preferred by anxious patients.
- If the pillow is removed to allow the patient to see outside the bore, consider using some support just under the neck.

## Sagittal

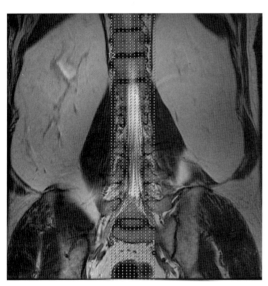

Figure 2.22 Sagittal planned on an axial image. (North Shore Radiology)

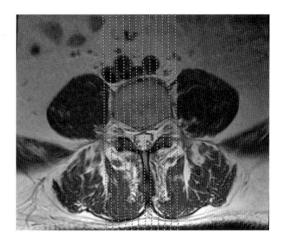

Figure 2.23 Sagittal planned on a coronal image. (North Shore Radiology)

## Alignment:

- Parallel to the long axis of the spinal cord.

## Coverage:

*Superior to inferior:*
- Conus to second sacral vertebra
- Coverage should include the twelfth thoracic vertebra, even if the conus is below this level

*Lateral to medial:*
- Vertebral pedicles on each side

*Posterior to anterior:*
- Spinous processes to prevertebral tissues.

## Demonstrates:

- Vertebral alignment, bony integrity and encroachment of retropulsed fragments on the canal in trauma
- Canal stenosis and lesions encroaching on the cauda equina
- End plate and cortical disruption, e.g. discitis
- Defects of the pars interarticularis +/− spondylo- or retro-listhesis
- Nerve root entrapment due to spondylolisthesis or lateral disc herniation
- Pseudomeningocele in the spinal foramina.

# Axial

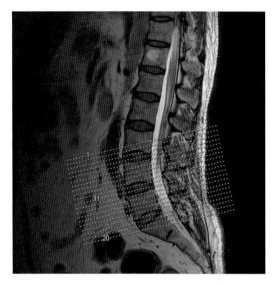

**Figure 2.24** Axial block series planned on a sagittal image.
(North Shore Radiology)

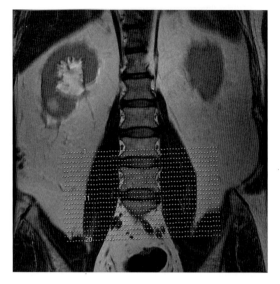

**Figure 2.26** Axial block series planned on a coronal image.
(North Shore Radiology)

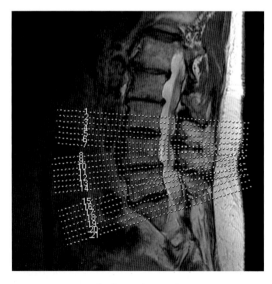

**Figure 2.25** Axial, planned to each intervertebral disc.
(North Shore Radiology)

## Alignment:

- Alignment may vary between sites. Two possibilities are available.
- As a single block:
  - in plane with the intervertebral discs.
- Using multiple angles:
  - aligned individually to each intervertebral disc space.
- Regardless of whether using a single block or multi-angle, slices should be aligned to the vertebral end plates in the coronal plane.

## Coverage:

*Superior to inferior:*
- Pedicle of the third lumbar vertebra to the pedicle of the first sacral segment for a single block, or from pedicle to pedicle for each individual vertebra.

- If lesions are evident higher, axial scans should also be performed through these levels.

*Lateral to medial:*
- Intervertebral foramina on each side

*Posterior to anterior:*
- Medial sacral crest to the prevertebral tissues.

## Demonstrates:

- Best plane for assessing disc impingement on spinal nerve roots
- Space-occupying lesions within the spinal canal
- Paravertebral extension of masses into the soft tissues
- Hypertrophy of the ligamentum flava.

# Imaging planes: Supplementary sequences

## Coronal

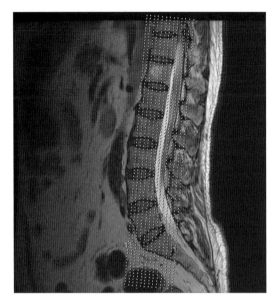

Figure 2.27 Coronal planned on a sagittal image.
(North Shore Radiology)

## Alignment:

- Parallel to the long axis of the cauda equina. Some obliquity will most likely be required to achieve this.

## Coverage:

*Superior to inferior:*
- Conus to second sacral vertebra
- Coverage should include the twelfth thoracic vertebra, even if the conus is tethered below this level

*Lateral to medial:*
- Transverse processes on each side

*Posterior to anterior:*
- Entire vertebral foramen to midway through the vertebral bodies.

## Demonstrates:

- Scoliosis
- Space-occupying lesions within the cauda equina
- Compression laterally on the nerve roots within the spinal foramina.

## Coronal oblique

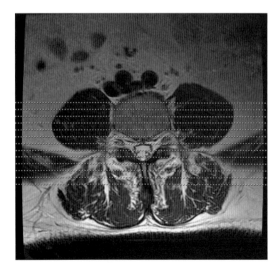

Figure 2.28 Coronal planned on an axial image.
(North Shore Radiology)

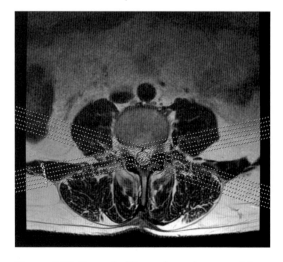

Figure 2.29 Coronal oblique planned on an axial image at the L3/4 level.
(North Shore Radiology)

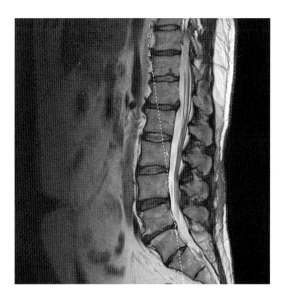

Figure 2.30 Coronal plane for demonstrating the nerve roots at the L3/4 level.
(North Shore Radiology)

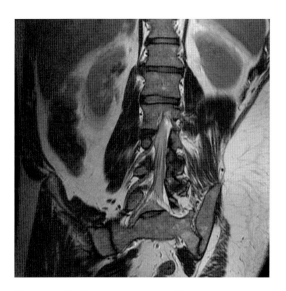

Figure 2.31 Right side coronal oblique image demonstrating L3/4 and L4/5 nerve roots exiting the foramina.
(North Shore Radiology)

## Alignment:

- Scans are targeted to the level clinically suspicious for disc herniation:
  - parallel to the nerve root on the suspicious side and disc level on an axial image
  - parallel to a line connecting the upper and lower end plates of the vertebrae above and below the disc level of interest on a mid-sagittal image.
- Bilateral scans may be performed simultaneously or separately. The plan demonstrates planning for both sides to be scanned together.

## Coverage:

*Superior to inferior:*
- Vertebrae immediately above and below the disc level of interest

*Lateral to medial:*
- Spinal nerve at the exit of the foramen to the cauda equina within the canal

*Posterior to anterior:*
- To cover the spinal foramen.

## Demonstrates:

- In plane demonstration of impingement of extra-foraminal disc lesions on nerve roots in the foramina.

# Chapter 2.4 Sacrum and coccyx

## Indications:

- Sacrococcygeal pain
- Sacroiliac joint pain or diastasis
- Arthritis (RA or OA)
- Malignancy, most frequently metastatic bone lesions
- Insufficiency fracture.

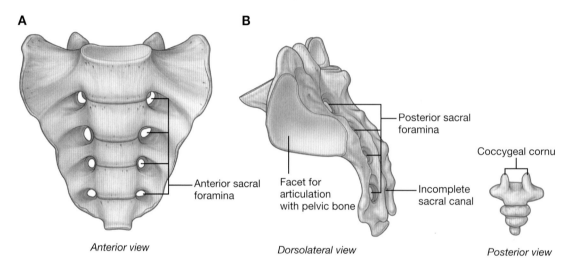

**A**       **B**

Anterior sacral foramina

Posterior sacral foramina

Coccygeal cornu

Facet for articulation with pelvic bone

Incomplete sacral canal

*Anterior view*       *Dorsolateral view*       *Posterior view*

Figure 2.32   An anterior view of the sacrum and a sagittal section A) and B).
(from Drake, Gray's Anatomy for Students 2e, with permission)

## Coils and patient considerations

The broad curved sacrum and coccyx form part of the pelvic girdle, as well as the lowest portion of the spine. The last intervertebral disc is found between the fifth lumbar vertebra and the first sacral segment. The spinal canal continues into the sacrum, the remaining cauda equina forming the five paired sacral and the single paired coccygeal nerves. There is no spinal canal within the coccyx.

Imaging of the sacrum and coccyx may be requested as part of the investigation of lower back pain or as an independent region. A similar imaging coil used for imaging the lumbar spine (Fig I.4) should provide sufficient coverage to include the most caudal coccygeal segments.

# Imaging planes: Routine sequences

## Position:

- Supine, head or feet first.

## Other considerations:

- Support the head with a pillow or sponges
- A feet-first orientation may be preferred by anxious patients
- If the pillow is removed to allow the patient to see outside the bore, consider using some support just under the neck.

# Coronal oblique

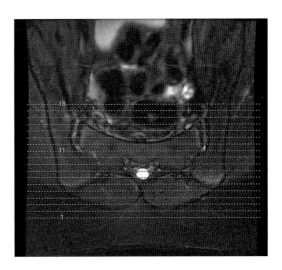

Figure 2.34  Coronal oblique planned on an axial image.
(North Shore Radiology)

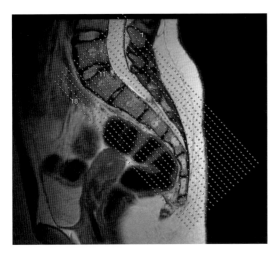

Figure 2.33  Coronal oblique planned on a sagittal image.
(North Shore Radiology)

## Alignment:

- Parallel to the long axis of the sacrum
- Parallel to a line connecting the posterior aspect of the sacroiliac joints.

## Coverage:

*Superior to inferior:*
- Superior end plate of the fifth lumbar vertebra to last coccygeal segment

*Lateral to medial:*
- Sacroiliac joints on each side

*Posterior to anterior:*
- Medial sacral crest to the anterior aspect of the fifth lumbar vertebra.

## Demonstrates:

- Fractures
- Bone lesions +/− cortical disruption
- Sacroiliac joint disruption or disease
- Sacral foramina and the exiting nerve roots.

# Axial oblique

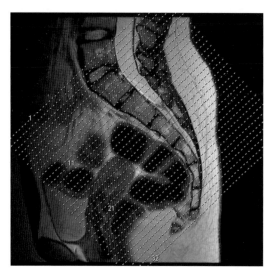

Figure 2.35 Axial oblique planned on a sagittal image.
(North Shore Radiology)

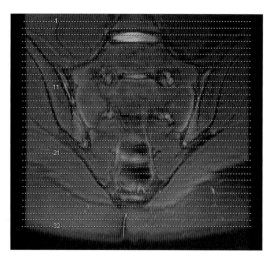

Figure 2.36 Axial oblique planned on a coronal image. (North Shore Radiology)

## Alignment:

· Perpendicular to the long axis of the sacrum
· Parallel to a line joining the superior aspect of the sacroiliac joints.

## Coverage:

· As per coronal oblique plane.

## Demonstrates:

· Sacroiliac joint disruption or disease.

# Imaging planes: Supplementary sequences

## Sagittal

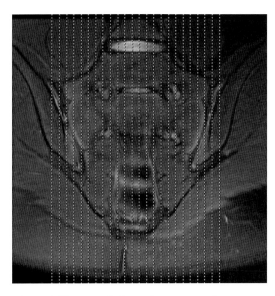

**Figure 2.37** Sagittal planned on a coronal image.
(North Shore Radiology)

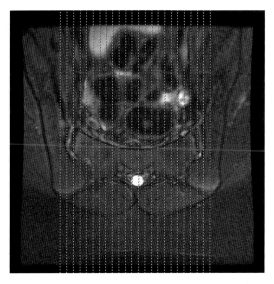

**Figure 2.38** Sagittal planned on an axial oblique image.
(North Shore Radiology)

## Alignment:

- Parallel to the long axis of the sacrum.

## Coverage:

*Superior to inferior:*
- Fifth lumbar vertebra to last coccygeal segment

*Lateral to medial:*
- Sacroiliac joints on each side

*Posterior to anterior:*
- Sacral processes to anterior border of fifth lumbar vertebra.

## Demonstrates:

- Fracture
- Spondylolisthesis of L5/S1
- Cortical expansion due to a benign or malignant lesion within the bone
- Cortical erosion due to invasion of a malignancy within the bone or the pelvic cavity.

# Chapter 2.5 Full spine

## Indications:

- Metastatic bone lesions or drop metastases
- Intramedullary cord lesions
- Suspected cord compression
- Juvenile scoliosis, associated with cord malignancies and syringomyelia and Chiari malformations, in isolation or in combination
- Neurofibromatosis.

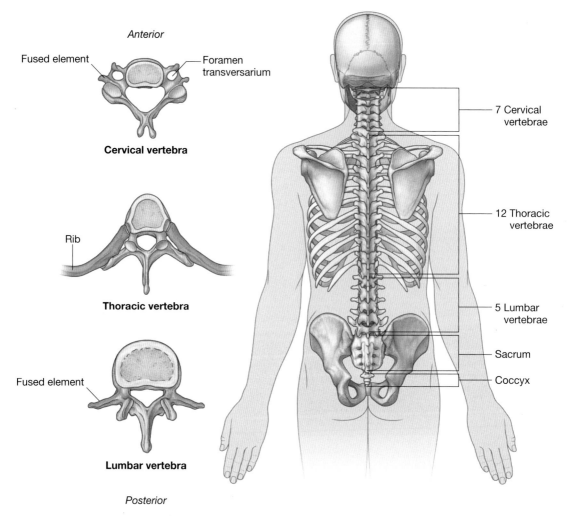

Figure 2.39 The vertebral column.
(from Drake, Gray's Anatomy for Students 2e, with permission)

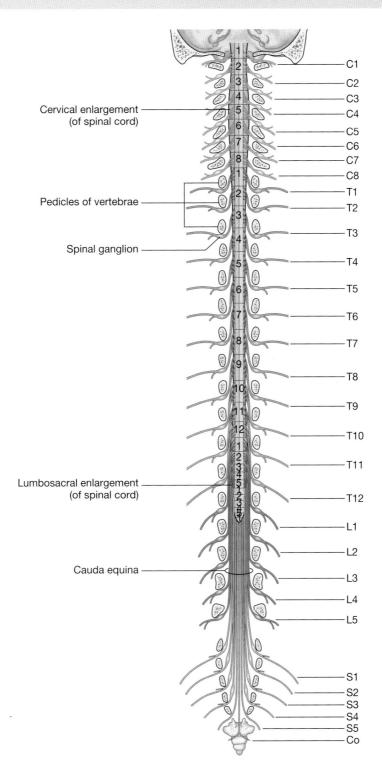

Figure 2.40 The relationships of the spinal nerve roots to the vertebrae.
(from Drake, Gray's Anatomy for Students 2e, with permission)

## Coils and patient considerations

Imaging of the entire spine is frequently requested in the assessment of suspected cord compression. This is a medical emergency, as prolonged compromise of neural function due to direct compression will result in irreversible neurological deficit. Patients suffering metastatic disease may not always be aware of the progression of disease; sudden loss of function or pain may be the first indication of severe disease. Determining the exact level of compression may not be easy as often multiple levels are affected. Full spine imaging may also be requested in the investigation of drop metastases and of scoliosis.

Image alignment for longer sagittal images follows similar principles to those described in Chapters 2.1 to 2.4. The main issue is to ensure all the vertebrae are imaged from the atlantooccipital joint to the sacrum. Axial scans are usually prescribed perpendicular to the spinal cord in regions suspicious for pathology, as directed by the supervising radiologist.

An imaging coil similar to that used for other regions of the spine is employed. Imaging is done in segments, and it is imperative to ensure that complete coverage is achieved without gaps. A method for ensuring this is described in Chapter 2.2 (Figs 2.12 & 2.13).

Patients suffering from severe scoliosis are not able to be imaged using long fields of view for sagittal images. Initially, coronal images using a long field of view should be taken. This will allow the operator to determine where the greatest changes in vertebral alignment occur and plan smaller sagittal segments. Three segments are generally sufficient. The important thing is to ensure that each and every vertebra is demonstrated. Axial scans are generally required at the points where the spinal canal or nerve root foramina are compromised by acute angulation between vertebrae. Image planning in this section demonstrates a technique for imaging the scoliotic spine.

# Imaging planes: Routine sequences

## Position:

- Supine, head first.

## Other considerations:

- Patients with severe scoliosis may require additional support with pads at some points along the spine, under the posterior ribs or the pelvis.

## Coronal

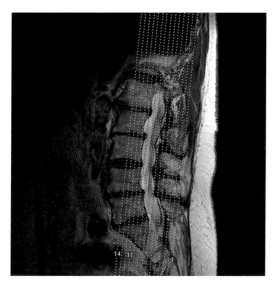

**Figure 2.41** Coronal lumbar spine planned on a sagittal image.
(North Shore Radiology)

## Alignment:

- Parallel to the long axis of the spinal cord. Some obliquity will most likely be required to achieve this.
- In conjunction with the scoliosis, vertebrae are often mal-rotated with respect to each other. Achieving alignment on axial images will generally require significant compromise.
- Planning is similar to other coronals (Chs 2.1–2.3).

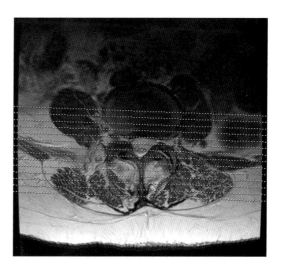

**Figure 2.42** Coronal lumbar spine planned on an axial image.
(North Shore Radiology)

## Coverage:

*Superior to inferior:*
- Atlantooccipital joint to fifth sacral segment, in two or three sections with overlap between each

*Lateral to medial:*
- Vertebral pedicles on each side. Extra slices may be required to ensure breadth of coverage at points of acute vertebral angulation

*Posterior to anterior:*
- Spinal processes to anterior vertebral bodies.

## Demonstrates:

- Scoliotic curves
- Likely lateral nerve root impingement at the points of greatest angulation between vertebrae
- Useful in helping establish vertebral levels through cross-referencing with other planes.

# Sagittal

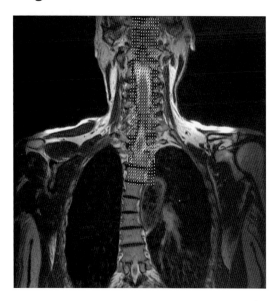

Figure 2.43 Sagittal cervical spine planned on a coronal image.
(North Shore Radiology)

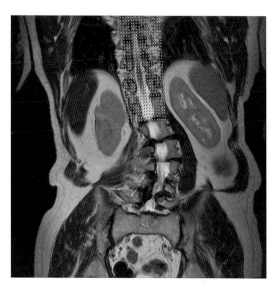

Figure 2.45 Sagittal thoracic spine planned on a coronal image of the lower spine. The coverage needs to be compared on a sagittal image higher up (see previous figure).
(North Shore Radiology)

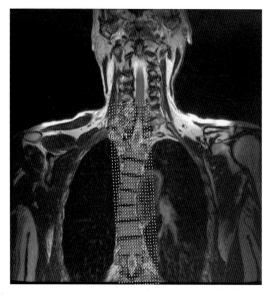

Figure 2.44 Sagittal thoracic spine planned on a coronal image of the upper spine. The coverage needs to be verified on a sagittal image lower down (see next figure).
(North Shore Radiology)

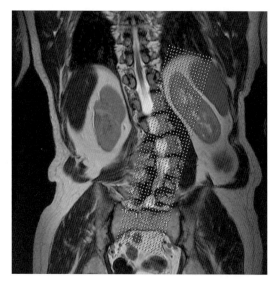

Figure 2.46 Sagittal lumbar spine planned on a coronal image.
(North Shore Radiology)

## Alignment:

- Parallel to the long axis of the spinal cord up to and including the vertebrae at the most acute angle of a scoliotic curve.
- Two or three segments may be required to cover the entire spine.

## Coverage:

*Superior to inferior:*
- Atlantooccipital joint to fifth sacral segment
- Scan in two or three segments with overlap

*Lateral to medial:*
- Transverse processes on each side

*Posterior to anterior:*
- Spinal processes to anterior vertebral bodies.

## Demonstrates:

- Chiari malformation at the base of skull
- Disc lesions
- Nerve root impingement.

# Axial

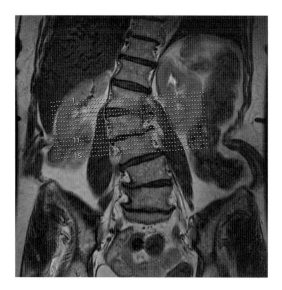

**Figure 2.47** Axial through the curvature planned on a coronal image.
(North Shore Radiology)

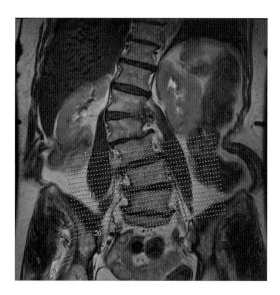

**Figure 2.48** A further set of axial scans planned through the lower lumbar vertebra.
(North Shore Radiology)

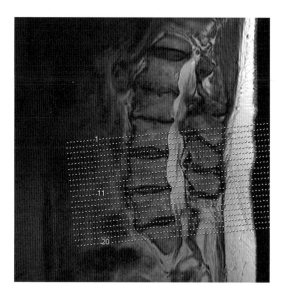

**Figure 2.49** Axial lower lumbar spine planned on a sagittal image.
(North Shore Radiology)

## Alignment:

- Perpendicular to the long axis of the spinal cord up to and including the vertebrae at a scoliotic curve.

## Coverage:

*Superior to inferior:*
- Determine the two vertebrae at the point of greatest acuteness
- Plan from the pedicle of the vertebra immediately above the start of the curve to the pedicle of the vertebra immediately below

*Lateral to medial:*
- Transverse processes on each side

*Posterior to anterior:*
- Spinal processes to anterior vertebral bodies.

## Demonstrates:

- Nerve root impingement at the most acute point, as well as the nerve roots immediately above and below
- Cord compromise.

# Further reading

Blake LC, Robertson WD, Hayes CE 1996 Sacral plexus: Optimal imaging planes for MR assessment. Radiology 199:767–772

Chi-Jen C, Hsu HL, Niu CC et al 2003 Cervical degenerative disease at flexion-extension MR imaging: Prediction Criteria. Radiology 227:136–142

Evans SC, Edgar MA, Hall-Craggs MA et al 1996 MRI of idiopathic juvenile scoliosis: A prospective study. Journal of Bone and Joint Surgery 78-B:314–317

Flannigan BD, Lufkin RB, McGlade C et al 1987 MR imaging of the cervical spine: Neurovascular anatomy. American Journal of Roentgenology 148:785–790

Goodman BS, Geffen JF, Mallempati S et al 2006 MRI images at a 45-degree angle through the cervical neural foramina: A technique for improved visualization. Pain Physician (9):327–332

Heo DH, Lee MS, Sheen SH et al 2009 Simple oblique lumbar magnetic resonance imaging technique and its diagnostic value for extraforaminal disc herniation. Spine 34(22):2419–2423

Jinkins JR, Matthes JC, Sener RN et al 1992 Spondylolysis, spondylolisthesis, and associated nerve root entrapment in the lumbosacral spine: MR evaluation. American Journal of Radiology 159:799–803

Larsson EM, Holtas S, Zygmunt S 1989 Pre- and postoperative MR imaging of the craniocervical junction in rheumatoid arthritis. American Journal of Roentgenology 152:561–566

Lee IS, Kim HJ, Lee JS et al 2009 Dural tears in spinal burst fractures: Predictable MR imaging findings. American Journal of Neuroradiology 30(1):14146

Parmar H, Park P, Brahma B et al 2008 Imaging of idiopathic spinal cord herniation. Radiographics 28:511–518

Reicher MA, Gold RH, Hallbach VV et al 1986 MR imaging of the lumbar spine: Anatomic correlations and the effects of technical variations. American Journal of Roentgenology 147:891–898

Udeshi U, Reeves D 1999 Routine thin slice MRI effectively demonstrates the lumbar pars interarticularis. Clinical Radiology 54:615–619

# Section 3

# Chest and abdomen

# Chapter 3.1 Mediastinum

## Indications:

- Mediastinal mass, e.g. thymic enlargement, lymphoma, congenital cysts.
- Neurogenic lesions, e.g. thoracic meningoceles, schwannomas, malignant nerve sheath tumours, sympathetic ganglia tumours.
- Differentiation between lymph nodes and vascular anomalies, particularly in patients

for whom iodinated contrast is contraindicated for CT.
- Assessment of vascular anomalies of the chest (in conjunction with MRA), e.g. thoracic aortic dissection or aneurysms.

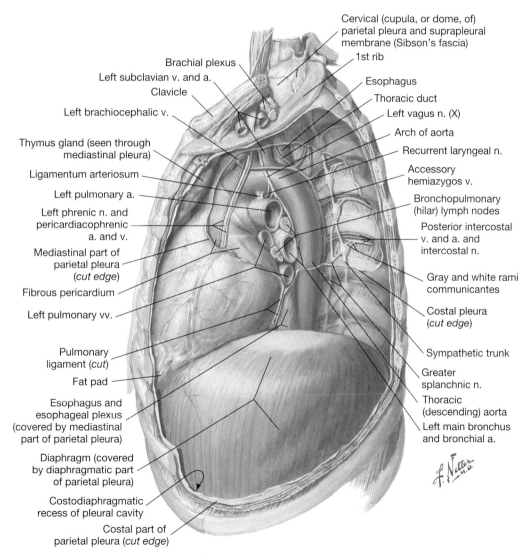

Figure 3.1 Divisions of the mediastinum.

# Coils and patient considerations

Contained within the chest between the pleurae and bounded anteroposteriorly by the sternum and thoracic vertebrae, the mediastinum refers to all the contents of the thoracic cavity except the lungs. Consensus for further division of the mediastinal compartments has been elusive, with some authors describing anterior, middle and posterior compartments. Other investigators describe a superior compartment with the inferior compartment being divided into three sections from anterior to posterior. Regardless of the morphologic convention employed, delineation of disease may include assessment of the heart, great vessels, thymus, trachea and left and right main bronchi, oesophagus, various nerves and lymph nodes.

The lack of signal-producing tissues in the lungs makes MRI an unsuitable technique for investigation of most pulmonary disorders, but it may be a useful adjunct for the demonstration of mediastinal lesions after CT or angiography. Lesions suspected to involve or originate in the spinal column often benefit from MRI in conjunction with CT to fully delineate disease pathogenesis. For patients who are subject to an increased lifetime accumulated risk of neoplastic disease due to breast or lung irradiation (e.g. young women with Hodgkin's lymphoma, lung cancer, breast cancer), MRI may be considered an appropriate alternative for monitoring of nodal disease, metastatic invasion to the heart or the investigation of cardiac function.

Inconsistent breath holds will limit image quality and potentially result in an incomplete examination. Respiratory gating used with free breathing techniques enables image triggering at a consistent point within the respiratory cycle. A respiratory bellows also allows the operator to monitor the patient's compliance with breath hold scans, alerting the operator to gradual exhalation during image acquisition or an inability to hold the breath for too long. It is useful to fit the bellows on every patient during preparation and to coach each one about breathing instructions before the examination. Advantage should be taken of options on scanners that facilitate pre-recorded breathing instructions.

Cardiac gating may also be useful, particularly for demonstration of the mediastinal lymph nodes close to the pericardium or thymus. While anatomic coverage in this section is quite broad, focus may be needed on a specific portion of the mediastinum. Direction from a radiologist should be sought to ensure the appropriate targeted examination is performed. A large area surface coil is required (see Figs I.1 & I.2).

# Imaging planes: Routine sequences

## Position:

- Supine, head first
- Arms above the head permits a smaller field of view for long axis imaging (coronal), as well as facilitating the examination of patients with a more solid body habitus.

## Other considerations:

- Patients who suffer from claustrophobia may prefer a feet-first orientation, if possible. Removing or using only a low pillow under the head may help the patient feel less encumbered, keeping distance between the face and top of the bore.
- The bellows should be positioned over the area of greatest expansion and contraction.
- If the bellows is positioned under the anterior portion of an imaging coil, consider placing the bellows along the side of the chest where the weight of the coil will not restrict its movement. Sponges or dielectric pads placed either side of the bellows also prevent the bellows from being compressed.

## Axial

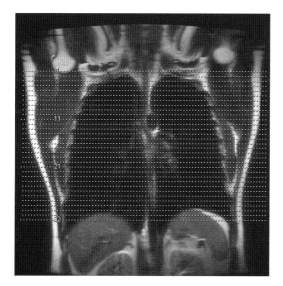

Figure 3.2 Axial planned on a coronal image.
(North Shore Radiology)

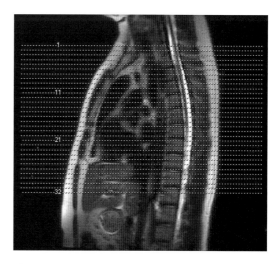

Figure 3.3 Axial planned on a sagittal image.
(North Shore Radiology)

## Alignment:

- True axial.

## Coverage:

*Superior to inferior:*
- Thoracic inlet to diaphragmatic crura

*Lateral to medial:*
- Chest wall on each side

*Posterior to anterior:*
- Thoracic spinous processes to sternum.

## Demonstrates:

- Contents of the mediastinum, comparative with direct acquisition CT images.
- Morphology of the great vessels and heart, with specific examination of each of the inferior mediastinal compartments.
- Lymph node location and size.

# Coronal

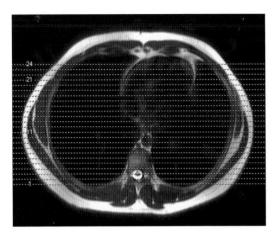

Figure 3.4 Coronal planned on an axial image.
(North Shore Radiology)

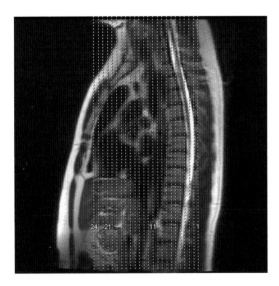

Figure 3.5 Coronal planned on a sagittal image.
(North Shore Radiology)

## Alignment:

- True coronal.

## Coverage:

- As for axial plane.

## Demonstrates:

- Contents of the mediastinum, comparable with reformatted CT images.
- Morphology of the great vessels and heart, with delineation of the superior and inferior mediastinal compartments.
- Lymph node location and size.
- Costophrenic angles and lung apices.

# Imaging planes: Supplementary sequences

## Sagittal

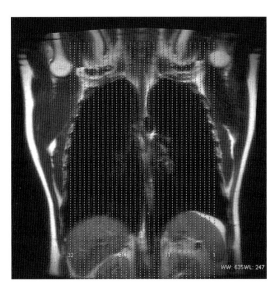

Figure 3.6 Sagittal planned on a coronal image.
(North Shore Radiology)

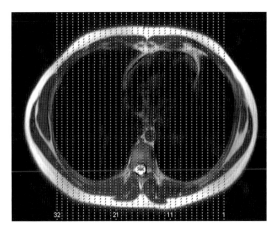

Figure 3.7 Sagittal planned on an axial image.
(North Shore Radiology)

## Alignment:

· True sagittal.

## Coverage:

· As for axial plane.

## Demonstrates:

· Contents of the mediastinum, comparable with reformatted CT images.
· Morphology of the great vessels and heart, with delineation of the superior and inferior mediastinal compartments.

# Chapter 3.2  Heart

## Indications:

- Benign cardiac mass, e.g. rhabdomyoma (generally paediatric only), myxoma, lipoma, fibroma.
- Primary cardiac malignancy, e.g. angiosarcoma, malignant fibrous histiocytoma (MFH), sarcoma, malignant paraganglioma, rhabdomyosarcoma (paediatric disease).
- Metastases from direct invasion of lung lesions or blood borne from other regions of the body.
- Thrombus.

## Coils and patient considerations

While the indications listed for this section focus on masses, imaging of the heart is performed for a much wider range of conditions, including myocardial infarction, pericarditis, and valvular and coronary disease. The imaging techniques and scan planes are complex. This section focuses on the basic imaging planes as they apply to assessment of gross cardiac anatomy and pathology. Comprehension of these initial planes places the student in good stead for progression to more involved clinical indications and morphologies at a later stage.

Imaging planes are described with relation to the chambers of the heart, rather than in relation to anatomical position. The base of the heart is high in the chest at the junction with the great vessels, with the apex inferior, above the diaphragm. Imaging of the heart requires a progressive approach, each plane planned from a previous. The long axis runs in plane with the cardiac septum. Imaging in plane with this long axis will provide a two-chamber view. A four-chamber view is created by planning scans perpendicular to the two-chamber view, the plane running from base to apex. Imaging perpendicular to both these planes produces short axis images. Planes are described in such a successive manner. All scans require ECG gating as well as patient compliance with holding the breath to ensure crisp anatomic detail by capturing images at the same point in the respiratory and cardiac cycles.

As for imaging of the mediastinum, a dedicated imaging coil such as those in Figures I.1 or I.2 is required.

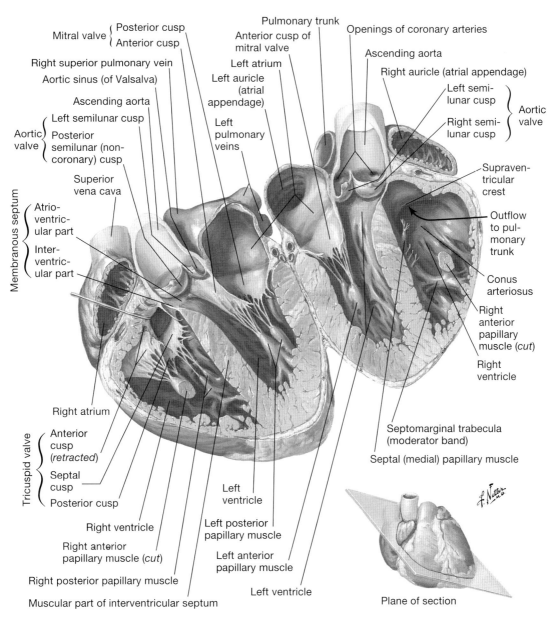

Figure 3.8 Ventricles and interventricular septum.
(Netter illustration from www.netterimages.com ©Elsevier Inc. All rights reserved.)

# Imaging planes: Routine sequences

## Position:

- Supine, head or feet first
- Arms above the head permits a smaller field of view for long axis imaging (coronal), as well as facilitating the examination of patients with a more solid body habitus.

## Other considerations:

- See Chapter 3.1.

## Two chamber

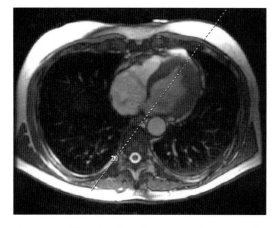

**Figure 3.9** Two-chamber view planned on an axial image.
(North Shore Radiology)

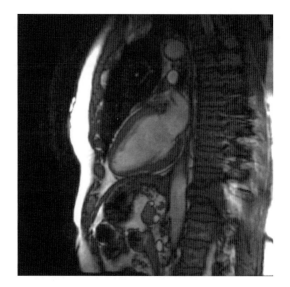

**Figure 3.10** Two-chamber image at end diastole.
(North Shore Radiology)

## Coverage:

*Superior to inferior:*
- Aortic bulb to the diaphragm

*Lateral to medial:*
- Usually a single slice through the midpoint of the left ventricle and atrium

*Posterior to anterior:*
- Vertebral bodies to apex of heart.

## Alignment:

- A plane passing through the apex of the heart to the midpoint of the mitral valve on an axial localiser image or four-chamber view, if available.

## Demonstrates:

- Generally a single slice T2 weighted cine SSFP image, demonstrating expansion and contraction of the left ventricle and atrium (LVLA) through one phase of the cardiac cycle.
- Masses within the chamber of the heart and their effect on valvular function.
- Useful for assessing abnormal wall motion.

# Short axis

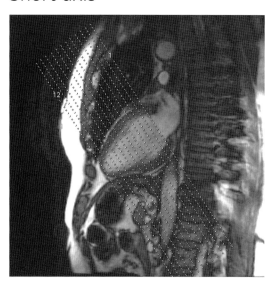

Figure 3.11 Short axis planned on a two-chamber view at end diastole.
(North Shore Radiology)

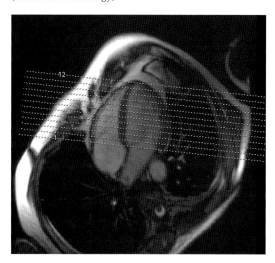

Figure 3.12 Short axis planned on a four-chamber view at end diastole.
(North Shore Radiology)

## Alignment:

- Select a two-chamber image at end diastole (when the chambers are fully relaxed and largest)

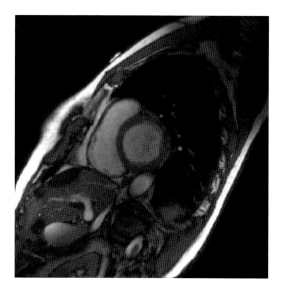

Figure 3.13 Short axis image at end diastole, through the left atrium and ventricle.
(North Shore Radiology)

- Position slices so the first slice is placed across the mitral valve annulus at end diastole.
- On a four-chamber view, the first slice should be across the mitral valve annulus at end diastole.

## Coverage:

*Superior to inferior:*
- Mitral valve to apex

*Lateral to medial:*
- Pericardium

*Posterior to anterior:*
- Apex of the heart to vertebral bodies.

## Demonstrates:

- Location of masses within the chambers of the heart and aspect of the wall to which they are attached
- Cardiac wall motion
- Used for calculation of ventricular volumes, mass and ejection fraction.

# Four chamber

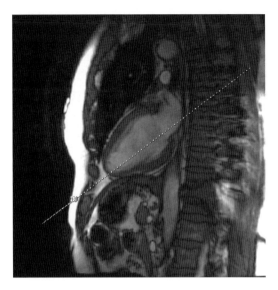

Figure 3.14  Four-chamber view planned on a
two-chamber image.
(North Shore Radiology)

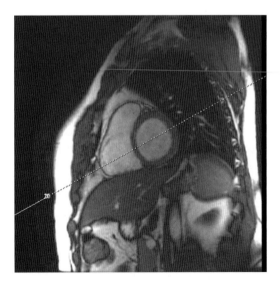

Figure 3.15  Four-chamber view planned on a short
axis image.
(North Shore Radiology)

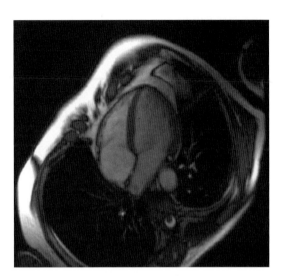

Figure 3.16  Four-chamber image.
(North Shore Radiology)

## Alignment:

- Use a two-chamber image at end diastole:
  - In a plane passing through the apex of the
    left ventricle and the mitral valve.
- Verified on a short axis image at end diastole:
  - Passing through the midpoint of the left
    ventricle and the apex of the heart. This will
    bisect the mitral and tricuspid valves and
    the interatrial septum.

## Coverage:

*Superior to inferior:*
- Mitral valve to apex

*Lateral to medial:*
- Pericardium

*Posterior to anterior:*
- Apex of the heart to vertebral bodies.

## Demonstrates:

- Location of masses within the chambers of the
  heart and aspect of the wall to which they are
  attached
- Impact of intra-chamber masses on cardiac
  motion and valvular function
- Cardiac wall motion.

# Coils and patient considerations

Suspended from the chest wall between the second and sixth ribs, the breast is attached to the pectoralis major and superior portion of the rectus abdominis muscles by a system of suspensory ligaments. Each breast is divided into a series of lobes, consisting of 15–25 milk-producing lobules. Ducts between each lobule carry milk to the nipple, which opens at the areola.

For high-risk carriers with the genetic markers BRCA1 and BRCA2, regular screening may be a normal part of life commencing when fibroglandular tissue is in abundance. The use of non-ionising technology addresses concerns about increasing the patient's lifetime accumulated risk of developing cancer due to incidental irradiation.

Mammography often encounters difficulties when examining the augmented breast, particularly in demonstrating lesions close to the chest wall. Ultrasound or MRI may be more successful in demonstrating pathology and also at examining the implant itself for structural damage.

Imaging coils are specially designed for breast imaging (Fig I.3). Symmetry is not always possible particularly in the post-surgical breast, but an effort should be made to minimise disparity as much as possible. Compression should be sufficient to stabilise tissue, but it is not intended to reduce width; density of tissue is not a factor for MRI.

Compression should not be so firm that tissue spills outside the imaging coil. Regardless of whether a breast implant is in situ or not, the glandular tissue must be encompassed in all planes and the implant, or extraneous silicone, must also be entirely covered.

Wherever possible, the arms should be raised above the head for imaging to reduce the field of view required and prevent aliasing in some planes. Imaging with one arm up and the other down may still allow a reduced field of view but will generally cause asymmetry, and should be discussed with the reporting radiologist before commencing.

Lesion detection and confirmation between datasets may be complicated by changes in tissue contours between sequences. Breast changes may be subtle, and in complex disease lesions can be confused if the patient moves. For studies in which subtraction of a pre-contrast dataset is performed from a dynamic contrast-enhanced dataset, the consequences of data misregistration cannot be overstated. Be sure your patient is comfortable, cannulated and reassured from the start to ensure a successful examination.

It must be remembered that a small percentage of breast cancers are actually in men, and that they too may be gene carriers. Although rare, these patients may be best imaged with a torso-type coil instead of a breast coil. A prone position will assist in managing respiratory motion.

# Imaging planes: Routine sequences

## Position:

- Prone, feet first
- Arms above the head permits a smaller field of view for long axis imaging (coronal), as well as facilitating the examination of patients with a more solid body habitus.

## Other considerations:

- Ensure the patient's head and neck are comfortable. Movement during scans can cause image blurring, while between datasets movement can result in misregistration.
- One or both arms down may be preferred for those who have pain from recent intervention or suffer shoulder pain.

## Axial

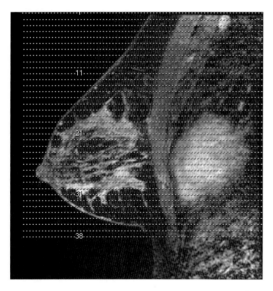

Figure 3.24 Axial breast with an implant planned on a sagittal image.
(North Shore Radiology)

## Alignment:

- True axial plane.

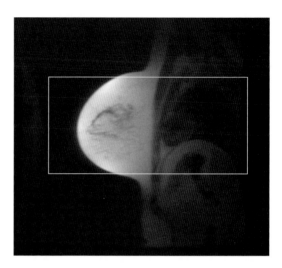

Figure 3.25 Axial volume of the breast, no implant, planned on a sagittal image.
(North Shore Radiology)

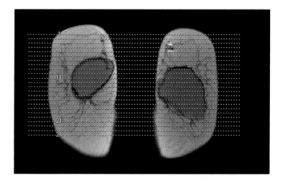

Figure 3.26 Axial breast with an implant planned on a coronal image.
(North Shore Radiology)

## Coverage:

*Superior to inferior:*
- Glandular tissue within the breast. Older women will have more fatty tissue
- For implants or intramammary silicone, coverage may need to extend further

*Lateral to medial:*
- Axillae on both sides

*Posterior to anterior:*
- Chest wall to nipples.

## Demonstrates:

- Relationship of lesions to the nipple, axillae and chest wall
- Often preferred for dynamic imaging as the total volume to be scanned is generally smallest in this plane
- Implants or silicone behind the pectoral muscle versus within the breast tissue.

# Sagittal: unilateral

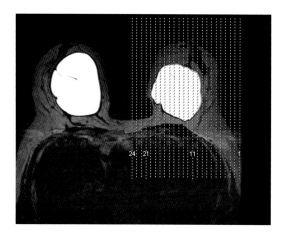

Figure 3.27 Sagittal breast with an implant planned on an axial image.
(North Shore Radiology)

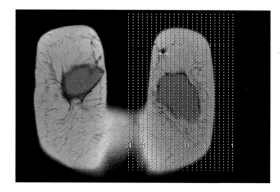

Figure 3.28 Sagittal breast with an implant planned on a coronal image.
(North Shore Radiology)

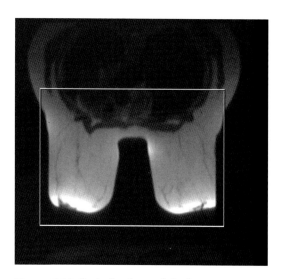

Figure 3.29 Sagittal volume of the breast, no impant, planned on an axial image.
(North Shore Radiology)

## Alignment:

- True sagittal plane
- Each breast may be scanned independently when temporal resolution is not an issue
- If dynamic imaging is performed in this plane, bilateral imaging may employ a single volume (Fig 3.28) or two volumes that run simultaneously.

## Coverage:

*Superior to inferior:*
- Manubrium of the sternum to most inferior aspect of breast

*Lateral to medial:*
- Axilla to sternum

*Posterior to anterior:*
- Chest wall to nipples.

## Demonstrates:

- Relationship of lesions to the nipple and chest wall
- An alternative plane for dynamic imaging.

# Coronal

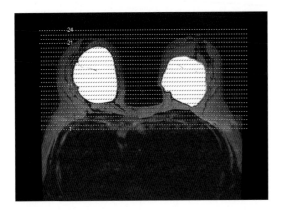

Figure 3.30 Coronal breast with an implant planned
on an axial image.
(North Shore Radiology)

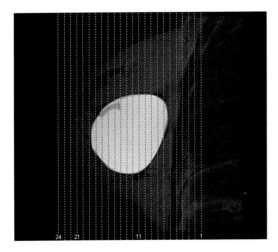

Figure 3.31 Coronal breast with an implant planned
on a sagittal image.
(North Shore Radiology)

## Alignment:

· True coronal plane.

## Coverage:

· As for axial plane.

## Demonstrates:

· Relationship of lesions to the axilla.

# Chapter 3.4  Liver and gall bladder

## Indications:

- Characterisation of lesions
  - Primary versus metastatic
  - Malignant versus benign
- Follicular nodular hyperplasia (FNH)
- Hepatocellular carcinoma (HCC)
- Haemangioma
- Hydatid cyst

- Metastatic spread
- Diffuse liver disease, e.g. haemochromatosis, cirrhosis
- Biliary obstruction, including choledocholithiasis
- Primary or secondary sclerosing cholangitis
- Cholangiocarcinoma.

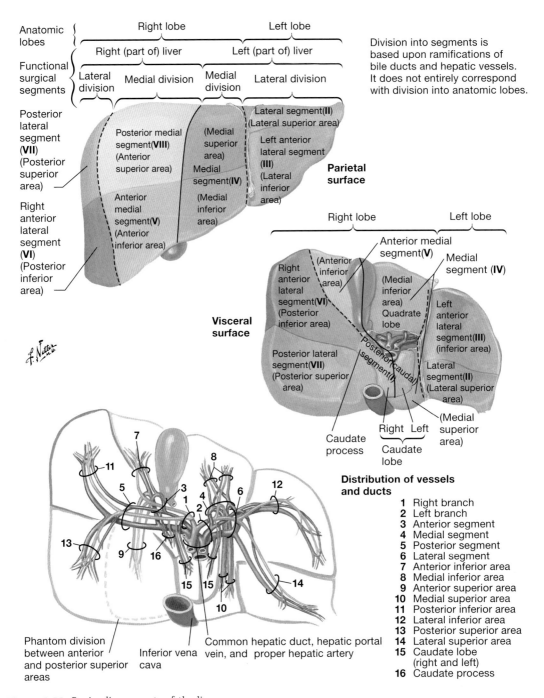

Division into segments is based upon ramifications of bile ducts and hepatic vessels. It does not entirely correspond with division into anatomic lobes.

**Distribution of vessels and ducts**

1  Right branch
2  Left branch
3  Anterior segment
4  Medial segment
5  Posterior segment
6  Lateral segment
7  Anterior inferior area
8  Medial inferior area
9  Anterior superior area
10 Medial superior area
11 Posterior inferior area
12 Lateral inferior area
13 Posterior superior area
14 Lateral superior area
15 Caudate lobe
   (right and left)
16 Caudate process

Figure 3.32 Couinad's segments of the liver.

(Netter illustration from www.netterimages.com ©Elsevier Inc. All rights reserved.)

# Coils and patient considerations

Located in the right upper quadrant of the abdomen, the liver is the second largest organ of the body, surpassed only by the skin. Situated immediately below the diaphragm, several systems exist for the discussion of anatomy of this organ; it is the physiological anatomy that is most crucial to the planning of surgical resection.

The liver receives blood from two sources. The common hepatic artery, originating at the coeliac trunk, feeds arterial blood to various organs in the upper abdomen. The gall bladder is fed by the cystic artery, and the liver by the left and right hepatic arteries.

Venous blood is supplied from the gastrointestinal tract via the main portal vein, entering the liver at the porta hepatis. This major vessel demarcates the line between the left and right lobes, supplying blood for both oxygenation and metabolic 'treatment' before venous drainage feeds into the inferior vena cava via the hepatic veins.

Eight segments are described according to Couinaud's classification. Segmentation of the superior segments from the inferior is delineated by the right and left portal veins. The right, middle and left hepatic veins comprise the venous drainage of the liver. When taken from their anastomosis with the IVC, they mark the longitudinal divisions between segments.

Bile produced in the liver collects in the canaliculi, feeding into the left and right biliary ducts. These anastomose to form the common hepatic duct before joining the cystic duct to form the common bile duct. Bile is stored in the gall bladder until required. When it contracts, bile passes through the continuation of the common bile duct reaching the ampulla of Vater at the junction with the pancreatic duct, before exiting through the sphincter of Oddi into the duodenum. In patients who have undergone cholecystectomy, bile drains freely. Common bile duct dimensions are 7–9 mm, depending on whether or not the patient has undergone cholecystectomy. Patients should fast for four hours prior to imaging to reduce secretions within the bowel and stomach that may impede diagnostic clarity and allow the gall bladder to fill. A large area surface coil is required (Figs I.1 & I.2).

# Imaging planes: Routine sequences

## Position:

- Supine, head or feet first
- Arms above the head is preferable as it permits a smaller field of view for long axis imaging (coronal), as well as facilitating the examination of patients with a more solid body habitus.

## Other considerations:

- As for Chapter 3.1
- Oral blueberry or pineapple juice may modify signal from gastrointestinal juices.

## Axial

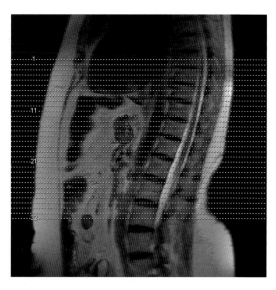

**Figure 3.34** Axial planned on a sagittal image. (North Shore Radiology)

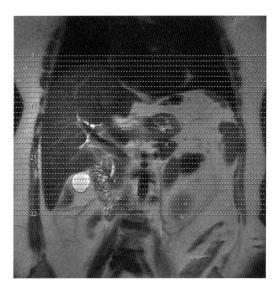

**Figure 3.33** Axial planned on a coronal image. (North Shore Radiology)

## Alignment:

- True axial plane.

## Coverage:

*Superior to inferior:*
- Dome of the liver to most inferior aspect of the tail of segment VI or the lowest border of the liver

*Lateral to medial:*
- Ribs on each side

*Posterior to anterior:*
- Peritoneum to anterior abdominal wall.

## Demonstrates:

- Individual inspection of liver segments
- Disruption of the biliary tree and vascular supply due to invasive disease
- Enables planning of multi-angle coronal oblique images for demonstration of the biliary tree (see Ch 3.4 Imaging planes: Supplementary sequences).

# Coronal

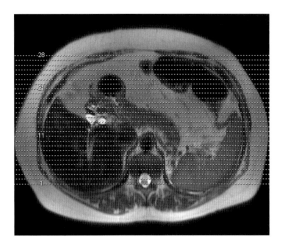

Figure 3.35 Coronal planned on an axial image.
(North Shore Radiology)

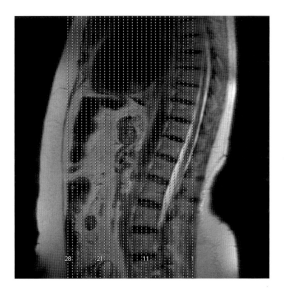

Figure 3.36 Coronal planned on a sagittal image.
(North Shore Radiology)

## Alignment:

- True coronal plane.

## Coverage:

*Superior to inferior:*
- Distal lung fields to tail of segment VI

*Lateral to medial:*
- Ribs on each side

*Posterior to anterior:*
- Peritoneum to anterior abdominal wall.

## Demonstrates:

- Lesions in the inferior tail and lateral tip of the left lobe
- Lesions high within the liver immediately under the diaphragm
- Confirms segmental orientation of lesions.

# Imaging planes: Supplementary sequences

## Coronal oblique (MR Cholangiopancreatography, MRCP)

Generally performed as a T2-weighted scan.

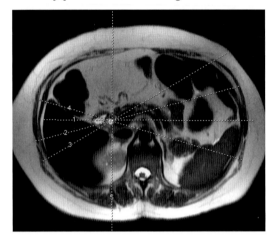

Figure 3.37 Multiple slices planned to bisect the CBD, including a sagittal slice. Figures 3.38 & 3.39 demonstrate the effect of altering the angle used.
(North Shore Radiology)

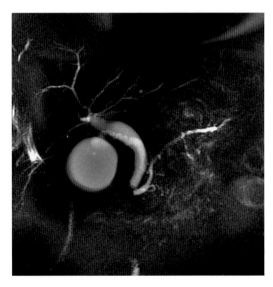

Figure 3.38 Coronal oblique image, demonstrating along the pancreatic duct, but barely separated from the CBD.
(North Shore Radiology)

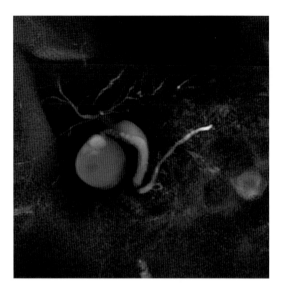

Figure 3.39 Coronal oblique image, demonstrating well separated ducts, but foreshortened pancreatic duct.
(North Shore Radiology)

## Alignment:

- Coronal plane and various angles either side
- A single thick cut, e.g. 50 mm, will generally image the entire biliary tree from porta hepatis to duodenum
- Individual body habitus affects ductal anatomy; angles of between 10° and 40° either side of the coronal plane may be required to separate the ductal anatomy
- More detailed information can be obtained by performing a stack of thin slices in the best plane.

## Coverage:

*Superior to inferior:*
- Dome of the liver to junction of the common bile duct with the duodenum

*Lateral to medial:*
- Full width of the liver

*Posterior to anterior:*
- Skin edge to skin edge.

## Demonstrates:

- High signal intensity of bile within the biliary and pancreatic ducts.
- Strictures evidenced by narrowing of the duct, as in sclerosing cholangitis.
- Dilatation of the biliary system due to increased pressure, the result of stenosis or obstruction.
  - Double duct sign, when both the pancreatic and common bile ducts are dilated and cease abruptly, is highly suggestive of malignancy in the ampulla or pancreatic head.
  - A hypointense signal within a duct may indicate introduced gas due to recent ERCP or a stone.
- Pancreas divisum (see Ch 3.6)
  - Isolated dilatation of the pancreatic duct in the tail, associated with pancreas divisum
  - Dual ducts within the pancreas.

# Chapter 3.5   Adrenals and kidneys

## Indications:

- Pheochromocytoma (PCC)
- Incidentaloma (mass found on another examination)
- Raised ACTH levels
- Cushing's syndrome (non-ACTH dependent; due to a non-pituitary cause)

- Adrenal adenoma or adrenocortical carcinoma (ACC)
- Renal cell cancer (RCC)
- Renal cyst
- Metastases
- Adrenal myelolipoma
- Von Hippel-Lindau disease.

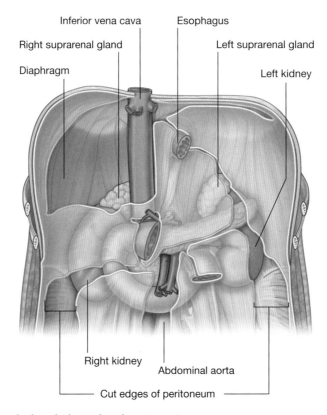

**Figure 3.40** Kidneys and adrenals, located in the retroperitoneum.
(From Drake, Gray's Anatomy for Students 2e, with permission)

# Coils and patient considerations

In the non-pathological examination, the paired adrenal glands are located superomedial to each kidney in the retroperitoneal space and weigh no more than 5 g. The adrenal on the right side is sandwiched between the diaphragmatic crus and the liver, almost immediately behind the inferior vena cava. Its counterpart on the left is more caudal, often seen at a level corresponding to the midpoint of the kidney on the right side. Both glands are offset anteromedially and superior to each kidney, and the fascia of the kidneys also envelops the adrenal glands. The kidneys are located between the twelfth thoracic and the third lumbar vertebrae.

Lesions of the adrenal gland are not uncommon, with as many as one in four cancer patients having metastases. Often an incidental lesion is discovered on other examinations. MRI is a useful adjunct to demonstrate lesion characteristics, particularly for pheochromocytoma, or for those with known hypersensitivity to iodinated contrast.

Highly mobile due to movement of the diaphragm, imaging must be performed with a breath-hold technique or respiratory triggering. Respiratory suspension is required to ensure complete examination. Consistency is the key to ensuring portions of the organs are not missed by suspending respiration at differing phases. It is highly recommended that patients be coached about holding the breath prior to commencing the examination.

It must be remembered that patients with renal impairment may not be suitable candidates for administration of gadolinium-based contrast. Be sure to check a recent creatinine level before discussing its use with the supervising radiologist. A large area surface coil similar to those used for abdominal imaging is required.

# Imaging planes: Routine sequences

## Position:

- Supine, head or feet first
- Arms above the head permit a smaller field of view for long axis imaging (coronal), as well as facilitating the examination of patients with a more solid body habitus.

## Other considerations:

- As for the liver (see Ch 3.4).

## Axial

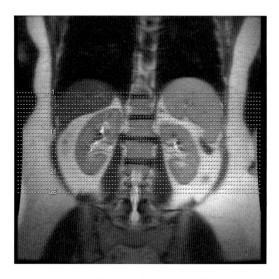

Figure 3.41 Axial planned on a coronal image. (North Shore Radiology)

## Alignment:

- True axial plane.

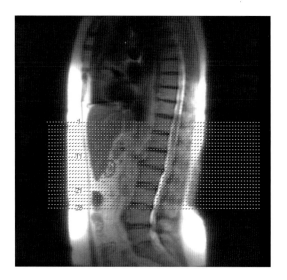

Figure 3.42 Axial planned on a sagittal image. (North Shore Radiology)

## Coverage:

*Superior to inferior:*
- Diaphragmatic crura to third lumbar vertebra

*Lateral to medial:*
- Ribs on each side

*Posterior to anterior:*
- Peritoneum to anterior abdominal wall.

## Demonstrates:

- Enlargement of the adrenal glands and/or kidneys
- Encroachment of masses on renal collecting system
- Relationship of lesions to surrounding structures.

# Coronal

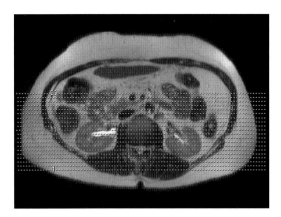

Figure 3.43  Coronal planned on an axial image.
(North Shore Radiology)

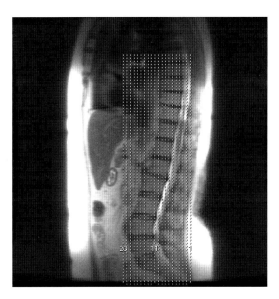

Figure 3.44  Coronal planned on a sagittal image.
(North Shore Radiology)

## Alignment:

- True coronal plane.

## Coverage:

*Superior to inferior:*
- Diaphragm to pelvic brim (iliac crests)

*Lateral to medial:*
- Ribs on each side

*Posterior to anterior:*
- Posterior ribs to anterior abdominal wall
- If lesions are known to be contained to the adrenal or kidney, coverage may be targeted from posterior ribs to mid-abdomen only.

## Demonstrates:

- Enlargement of the adrenal glands and/or kidneys
- Better than axial for evaluation of disease invasion into surrounding structures, especially IVC
- Lesions within the poles of the kidneys.

# Imaging planes: Supplementary sequences

## Sagittal

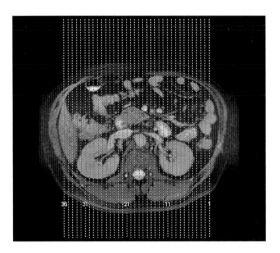

Figure 3.45  Sagittal planned on an axial image.
(North Shore Radiology)

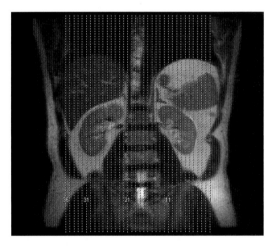

Figure 3.46  Sagittal planned on a coronal image.
(North Shore Radiology)

## Alignment:

• True sagittal plane.

## Coverage:

*Superior to inferior:*
• Diaphragm to pelvic brim (iliac crests)

*Lateral to medial:*
• Renal fascia on each side

*Posterior to anterior:*
• Posterior ribs to anterior abdominal wall.

## Demonstrates:

• Enlargement of the adrenal glands and/or kidneys
• Better than axial for evaluation of disease extension into IVC
• Lesions within the poles of the kidneys.

# Chapter 3.6  Pancreas

## Indications:

- Pancreatic cancer
- Pancreatitis, acute or chronic
- Pancreas divisum

- Annular pancreas
- Pancreatic duct stones
- Metastases.

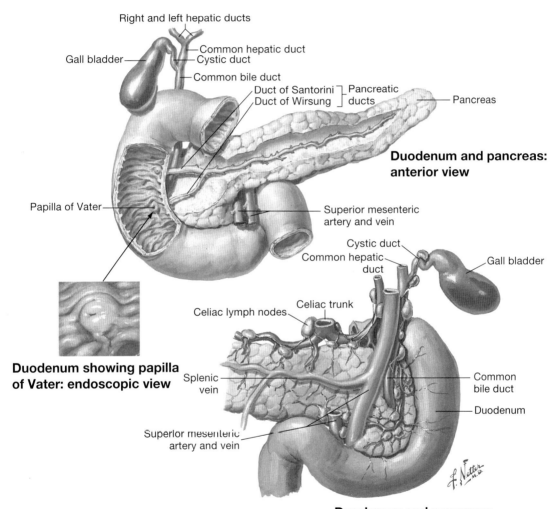

Figure 3.47  Anatomy of the pancreas.
(Netter illustration from www.netterimages.com ©Elsevier Inc. All rights reserved.)

## Coils and patient considerations

Deep within the abdomen, the tail of this retroperitoneal organ begins anterior to the first lumbar vertebra. It extends posteroinferiorly beneath the stomach and across the midline, before the head and uncinate process nestles into the curve of the duodenum. The pancreatic duct (duct of Wirsung) extends from tail to head up to 17 cm in length, exiting at the major papilla and merging with the common bile duct to form the ampulla of Vater. The normal pancreatic duct should be no more than 3 mm in diameter.

Anomalous morphology can develop during gestation, resulting in pancreas divisum. This potentially problematic condition may impact on pancreatic drainage, increasing the risk of pancreatitis and complicate surgery. In rare cases of annular pancreas in which the pancreas partially or completely encircles the duodenum, a third duct persists communicating with the CBD or the duct of Wirsung.

Patients suffering from pancreatic disease often suffer acute or chronic pancreatitis causing obstruction, inducing intense pain in the back. Demonstration of pathology may be difficult if the ducts are not significantly dilated. Administration of intravenous secretin improves visualisation of ductal morphology with peak dilatation achieved about 5 minutes after administration. The underlying clinical indication will direct the radiologist's decision on its use.

All patients attending for abdominal imaging should fast for at least four hours prior to imaging to reduce secretions within the bowel and stomach that may impede diagnostic clarity and to allow the gall bladder to fill. As with imaging of the gall bladder, oral contrast may be used (Ch 3.4).

Imaging coils used are similar to those for all chest and abdomen scanning; a large field of view being necessary to ensure that not only the pancreas is imaged but also any potential invasion of adjacent structures. Management of respiratory motion is essential, using respiratory triggering with a bellows or by a breath-hold technique, as discussed in earlier chapters.

# Imaging planes: Routine sequences

## Position:

- Supine, head or feet first
- Arms above the head permit a smaller field of view for long axis imaging (coronal), as well as facilitating the examination of patients with a more solid body habitus.

## Other considerations:

- As for the liver (chapter 3.4)

## Axial

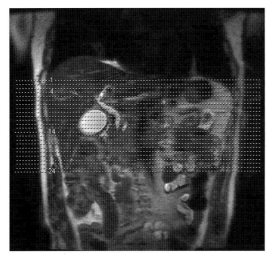

Figure 3.48  Axial planned on a coronal image. (North Shore Radiology)

## Alignment:

- True axial plane.

## Coverage:

*Superior to inferior:*
- Eleventh thoracic to third lumbar vertebrae
- For adenocarcinoma (to enable staging), dome of the diaphragm to third lumbar vertebra or inferior tip of the liver, whichever extends more inferiorly

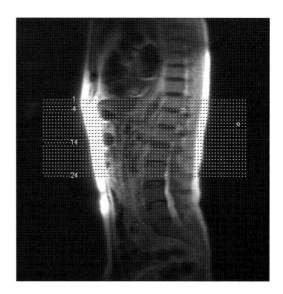

Figure 3.49  Axial planned on a sagittal image. (North Shore Radiology)

*Lateral to medial:*
- Ribs on each side

*Posterior to anterior:*
- Posterior to anterior abdominal walls.

## Demonstrates:

- Enlargement of the pancreas, particularly the head
- Encroachment of masses on the renal collecting system
- Relationship of lesions to surrounding structures, particularly the duodenum, common bile duct and ampulla
- Clarify organ morphology in cases of suspected pancreas divisum or annular pancreas.

# Coronal

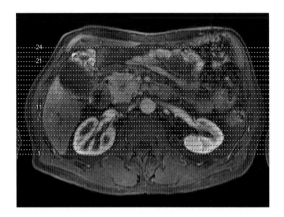

Figure 3.50  Coronal planned on an axial image.
(North Shore Radiology)

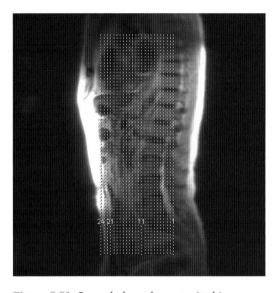

Figure 3.51  Coronal planned on a sagittal image.
(North Shore Radiology)

## Alignment:

- True coronal plane.

## Coverage:

*Superior to inferior:*
- Diaphragm to pelvic brim (iliac crests)

*Lateral to medial:*
- Ribs on each side

*Posterior to anterior:*
- Posterior to anterior abdominal walls.

## Demonstrates:

- Enlargement of the pancreas
- Dilatation of the common bile and intrahepatic ducts.

Imaging planes: Supplementary sequences

## Coronal oblique (MR Cholangiopancreatography, MRCP)

Refer to Chapter 3.5 Imaging planes: Supplementary sequences.

# Chapter 3.7  Aorta

## Indications:

- Vascular occlusion
- Claudication
- Stenosis
- Aneurysm

- Dissection
- Arteriovenous malformation
- Congenital anomalies.

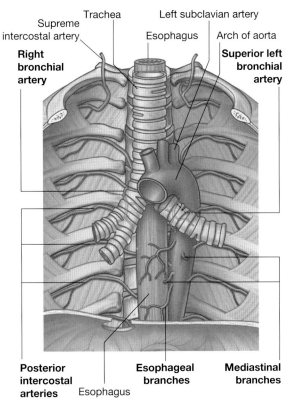

Trachea
Left subclavian artery
Supreme intercostal artery
Esophagus
Arch of aorta
**Right bronchial artery**
**Superior left bronchial artery**
**Posterior intercostal arteries**
Esophagus
**Esophageal branches**
**Mediastinal branches**

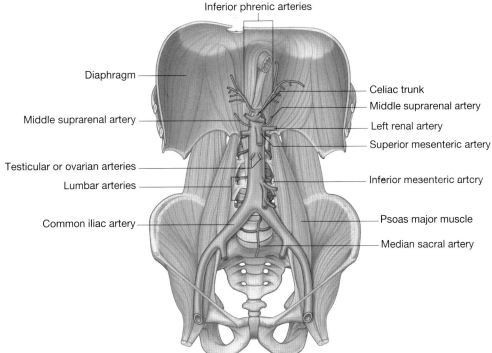

Inferior phrenic arteries
Diaphragm
Middle suprarenal artery
Testicular or ovarian arteries
Lumbar arteries
Common iliac artery
Celiac trunk
Middle suprarenal artery
Left renal artery
Superior mesenteric artery
Inferior mesenteric artery
Psoas major muscle
Median sacral artery

Figure 3.52 Branches originating from the aorta.
(From Drake, Gray's Anatomy for Students 2e, with permission)

# Coils and patient considerations

Commencing with the ascending portion at the aortic valve, the aorta is the largest vessel in the body. The left and right coronary arteries arise just after the aortic root. The characteristic 'candy cane' curve formed by the aortic arch gives rise to the vessels feeding the head and neck. While many possible anomalous variations exist, the three major branches are the left common carotid, left subclavian and the innominate arteries. The peak of the arch is generally about 2.5 cm below the manubrium.

Continuing caudally, the descending or thoracic aorta commences at the level of the fourth thoracic vertebra, beginning left of the spine and gradually moving to sit directly anterior. At the aortic hiatus in the diaphragm at the level of the twelfth thoracic vertebra, it becomes known as the abdominal aorta.

The coeliac axis, a short 'stump' giving rise to the splenic, hepatic and left gastric arteries, is the first branch arising from the abdominal aorta, just below the diaphragm at the level of the twelfth thoracic vertebra. Like the coeliac axis, the superior and inferior mesenteric arteries are unpaired, all arising from the anterior aspect of the aorta. The superior and inferior mesenteric arteries arise at the level of the first and third lumbar vertebrae, respectively.

The paired small suprarenal arteries feed the adrenals, arising from the lateral aspect of the aorta at the level of the first lumbar vertebra, just above the renal arteries. The thin gonadal arteries (internal spermatic arteries in men, ovarian arteries in women) also arise in pairs, but from the posterior aspect of the aorta, at the level of the second lumbar vertebra. Finally, the aorta divides to create the left and right common iliac arteries in front of the body of the fourth lumbar vertebra.

Anomalous development of the aorta can result in a range of congenital problems. Often patients will have had other imaging, with the MR examination forming part of a comprehensive pre-surgical assessment or follow-up.

In the examination of acquired disease, MRI may be used in conjunction with computed tomography, digital subtraction angiography or independently. It must be borne in mind that for some conditions, such as aortic dissection, it may be necessary to extend imaging beyond the anatomic limits of the thorax, abdomen or pelvis to demonstrate the true extent of pathology. Baseline axial scans determining gross pathology may be prescribed initially by a supervising radiologist, allowing further scans to be targeted as required.

Gating with ECG provides the best quality images of the ascending aorta and the arch, with respiratory gating or image acquisition on suspended respiration further improving image quality. It is prudent to use an imaging coil designed for imaging of the heart when available (Figs I.1 & I.2). Otherwise, a large field of view coil should provide good signal. Raw data should always be provided to the reporting radiologist, along with maximum intensity projections or surface rendered images, to ensure pathology is not missed (Fig 3.53). Plans in this section assume the use of a gadolinium-based contrast medium.

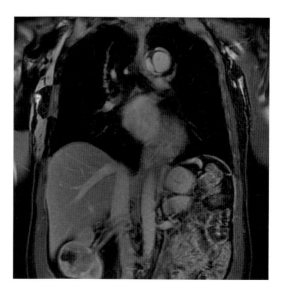

Figure 3.53 A dissected aortic arch, demonstrated on the raw data. This lesion was not readily apparent on the maximum intensity projection (see Fig 3.55). (Midland MRI)

# Imaging planes: Routine sequences

## Position:

- Supine, head or feet first
- Arms above the head is preferable as it permits a smaller field of view for long axis imaging (coronal), as well as facilitating the examination of patients with a more solid body habitus.

## Other considerations:

- As for liver (Ch 3.4).

## Sagittal oblique: thoracic aorta

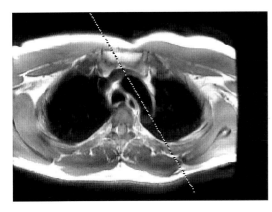

Figure 3.54 Sagittal oblique plane on an axial image.
(North Shore Radiology)

## Alignment:

- In plane with the aortic arch on an axial image.

## Coverage:

*Superior to inferior:*
- Origins of neck vessels to aortic bifurcation is ideal, especially for investigation of dissection, but may be limited by the field of view
- Try to include the origin of the renal arteries if signal coverage is limited

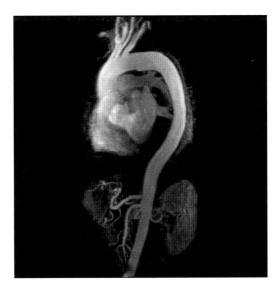

Figure 3.55 Sagittal oblique MIP through the thoracic aorta.
(Midland MRI)

*Lateral to medial:*
- Cardiac borders and renal arteries on each side

*Posterior to anterior:*
- Posterior chest wall (thoracic aorta) to left atrium.

## Demonstrates:

- Origins of the arteries of the neck
- Morphology of the ascending and descending aorta and the arch.

# Coronal: abdominal aorta

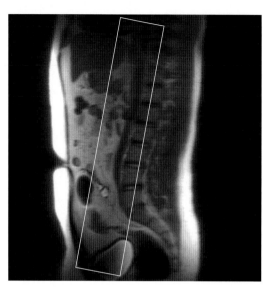

Figure 3.56 Coronal oblique planned on a sagittal image.
(North Shore Radiology)

## Alignment:

- Parallel to the long axis of the thoracic aorta.

## Coverage:

*Superior to inferior:*
- Domes of the diaphragm to common iliac artery bifurcations

*Lateral to medial:*
- Renal arteries and common iliac artery bifurcations

*Posterior to anterior:*
- Posterior renal capsule to mid-pancreas and bifurcation of common iliac arteries.

## Demonstrates:

- Patency of abdominal aorta and branches
- Length and degree of stenotic sections of vessels
- Development of enlarged collateral circulation.

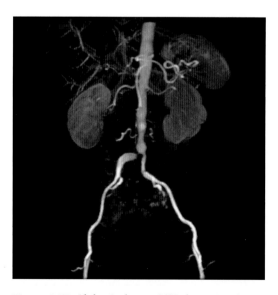

Figure 3.57 Abdominal aorta MIP, demonstrating stenosis at the aortic bifurcation.
(Midland MRI)

# Further reading

Ahualli J 2007 The double duct sign. Radiology 244(1):314–315

Baumgarten DA, Smith JK, Kenney P 2009 Renal cell carcinoma. emedicine. Online. Available: http://emedicine.medscape.com/article/380543-print, 14 Mar 2011

Boiselle PM, Patz EF, Vining DJ et al 1998 Imaging of mediastinal lymph nodes: CT, MR, and FDG PET. Radiographics 18(5):1061–1069

Causer PA, Jong RA, Warner E et al 2007 Breast cancers detected with imaging screening in the BRCA population: Emphasis on MR Imaging with histopathologic correlation. Radiographics 27(S1):S165–S182

Chalazonitis NA, Lachanis BS, Laspas F et al 2008 Pancreas divisum: Magnetic resonance cholangiopancreatography findings. Singapore Medical Journal 49(11):951–954

Eccles DA 2008 Identification of personal risk of breast cancer: Genetics. Breast Cancer Research 10(S4):S12

Ernst O, Asselah T, Sergent G et al 1998 MR cholangiography in primary sclerosing cholangitis. American Journal of Roentgenology 171(4):1027–1030

Ferguson EC, Krishnamurthy R, Oldham SA 2007 Classic imaging signs of congenital cardiovascular abnormalities. Radiographics 27(5):1323–1334

Fukukura Y, Fujiyoshi F, Sasaki M et al 2002 Pancreatic duct: Morphologic evaluation with MR cholangiopancreatography after secretin stimulation. Radiology 222:674–680

Fulcher AS, Turner MA 1999 MR pancreatography: A useful tool for evaluating pancreatic disorders. Radiographics 19(1):5–24

Graziani R, Tapparelli M, Malago R et al 2005 The various imaging aspects of chronic pancreatitis. Journal of the Pancreas 13:6(1S):73–88

Juergens U, Fischbach R 2005 Multidetector-row CT assessment of left-ventricular function. In: Schoepf UJ (ed.) CT of the Heart. Humana, New Jersey, 183–194

Kandpal H, Bhatia V, Garg P et al 2009 Annular pancreas in an adult patient: Diagnosis with endoscopic ultrasonography and magnetic resonance cholangiopancreatography. Singapore Medical Journal 50(1):e29–e31

Kay SM, Flageole H 2008 Adrenal glands. emedicine. Online. Available: http://emedicine.medscape.com/article/940347-print, 14 Mar 2011

Khan MA, Akhtar I 2010 Pancreas divisum. emedicine. Online. Available: http://emedicine.medscape.com/article/371511-print, 14 Mar 2011

Kim TK, Kim BS, Kim JH et al 2002 Diagnosis of intrahepatic stones: Superiority of MR cholangiopancreatography over endoscopic retrograde cholangiopancreatography. American Journal of Roentgenology 179:429–434

Krishnan A, Shirkhoda A 2010 Pheochromocytoma. emedicine. Online. Available: http://emedicine.medscape.com/article/379861-print, 14 Mar 2011

Kuhl C 2007 The current status of breast MR imaging, Part I: Choice of technique, image interpretation, diagnostic accuracy and transfer to clinical practice. Radiology 244(3):356–378

Layton KF, Kallmes DF, Cloft HJ et al 2006 Bovine aortic arch variant in humans: Clarification of a common misnomer. American Journal of Neuroradiology 26:1541–1542

Lee VS 2002 Cardiac MRI: Practical protocols and cases. Medscape Today. Online. Available: http://www.medscape.com/viewarticle/432905_4, 14 Mar 2011

Mader MT, Poulton TB, White RD 1997 Malignant tumors of the heart and great vessels: MR imaging appearance. Radiographics 17(1):145–153

Mansmann G, Lau J, Balk E et al 2004 The clinically inapparent adrenal mass: Update in diagnosis and management. Endocrine Reviews 25(2):309–340

Martin DR, Semelka RD 2007 Health effects of ionizing radiation from diagnostic CT imaging: Consideration of alternative imaging strategies. Applied Radiology 36(6)

Miller FH, Rini NJ, Keppke AL 2006 MRI of adenocarcinoma of the pancreas. American Journal of Roentgenology 187(4):W365–W374

Papanikolaou N, Karantanas A, Maris T et al 2000 MR cholangiopancreatography before and after oral blueberry juice administration. Journal of Computer Assisted Tomography 24(2):229–234

Reinhold C, Bret PM, Guibald L et al 1996 MR cholangiopancreatography: Potential clinical applications. Radiographics 16(2):309–320

Restrepo CS, Eraso A, Ocazionez D et al 2008 The diaphragmatic crura and retrocrual space: Normal imaging appearance, variants and pathologic conditions. Radiographics 28(5):1289–1305

Riordan RD, Khonsari M, Jeffries J et al 2004 Pineapple juice as a negative oral contrast agent in magnetic resonance cholangiopancreatography: A preliminary evaluation. British Journal of Radiology 77(924):991–999

Rutkauskas S, Gedrimas V, Pundzius J et al 2006 Traditional surgical viewpoint of liver anatomy and definition of the Couinaud segments. Medicina 42(2)98–106

Sadhev A, Reznek RH, Evanson J et al 2007 Imaging in Cushing's Syndrome. Arquivos Brasileiros de Endocrinologia e Metabologia 51(8):1319–1328

Smithius R 2006 Liver: Segmental anatomy. In: The Radiology Assistant. 7 May. Online. Available: http://www.radiologyassistant.nl/en/4375bb8dc241d#, 14 Mar 2011

Sparrow PJ, Kurian JB, Jones TR et al 2005 MR imaging of cardiac tumors. Radiographics 25(5):1255–1276

Strollo DC, Rosado-de-Christenson ML, Jett JR 1997 Primary mediastinal tumors: Part I Tumors of the anterior mediastinum. Chest 112(2):511–522

Strollo DC, Rosado-de-Christenson ML, Jett JR 1997 Primary mediastinal tumors: Part II Tumors of the middle and posterior mediastinum. Chest 112:1344–1357

Strunk H [no date] Limitations and pitfalls of Couinaud's segmentation of the liver in transaxial imaging. Universitat Bonn. Online. Available: http://www.uni-bonn.de/~umm705/quiz0403.htm, 14 Mar 2011

Turner MA, Fulcher AS 2001 The cystic duct: Normal anatomy and disease processes. Radiographics 21(1):3–22

Varghese A 2008 Principles of CMR. In: Varghese A, Pennel DJ (eds) Cardiovascular magnetic resonance made easy. Churchill Livingstone, Edinburgh, 1–20

Ward J, Sheridan MB, Guthrie JA et al 2004 Bile duct strictures after hepatobiliary surgery: Assessment with MR Cholangiography. Radiology 231(1):101–108

Yu J, Turner MA, Fulcher AS et al 2006 Congenital anomalies and normal variants of the pancreaticobiliary tract and the pancreas in adults: Part 2 Pancreatic duct and pancreas. American Journal of Roentgenology 187(6):1544–1553

Zidi SH, Prat F, Le Guen O et al 1999 Use of magnetic resonance cholangiography in the diagnosis of choledocholithiasis: prospective comparison with a reference imaging method. Gut 44(1):118–122

# Section 4

# Pelvis

# Chapter 4.1  Rectum and anus

## Indications:

- Rectal carcinoma
- Ulcerative colitis, Crohn's disease
- Pre-sacral abscess
- Congenital malformations

- Endometriosis
- Extension of disease from other pelvic organs
- Fistula-in-ano.

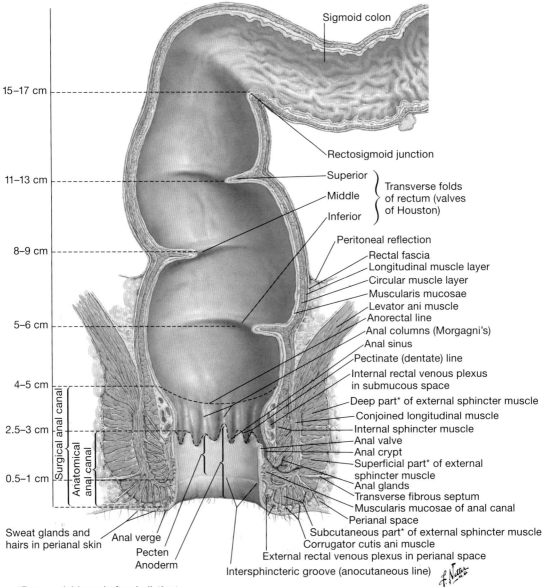

Sigmoid colon

15–17 cm

11–13 cm

8–9 cm

5–6 cm

4–5 cm

2.5–3 cm

0.5–1 cm

Surgical anal canal

Anatomical anal canal

Rectosigmoid junction

Superior
Middle
Inferior

Transverse folds of rectum (valves of Houston)

Peritoneal reflection
Rectal fascia
Longitudinal muscle layer
Circular muscle layer
Muscularis mucosae
Levator ani muscle
Anorectal line
Anal columns (Morgagni's)
Anal sinus
Pectinate (dentate) line
Internal rectal venous plexus in submucous space
Deep part* of external sphincter muscle
Conjoined longitudinal muscle
Internal sphincter muscle
Anal valve
Anal crypt
Superficial part* of external sphincter muscle
Anal glands
Transverse fibrous septum
Muscularis mucosae of anal canal
Perianal space
Subcutaneous part* of external sphincter muscle
Corrugator cutis ani muscle
External rectal venous plexus in perianal space

Sweat glands and hairs in perianal skin
Anal verge
Pecten
Anoderm
Intersphincteric groove (anocutaneous line)

*Parts variable and often indistinct

Figure 4.1  The rectum & anus.

# Coils and patient considerations

Located at the level of the third sacral vertebra, the rectosigmoid junction marks the end of the absorptive portion of the gastrointestinal tract, the rectum itself serving as a storage point for faeces. Transition between the rectum and anus extends approximately 1.5 cm, marked by the columns of Morgagni, before the gastrointestinal tract terminates at the anal verge 2–4 cm distally.

The rectum follows the sacrococcygeal curve contained within the mesorectal fat, which in turn is surrounded by the mesorectal fascia. Within the fat are lymph nodes, vessels and nerves servicing the rectum and other pelvic organs. The proximal two-thirds of the rectum are within the peritoneal cavity, the inferior aspect of which is marked by the levator ani, the marker of the anorectal junction. Demonstration of tumour extension beyond the mesorectal fascia helps establish disease stage and appropriate treatment.

The internal and external anal sphincters control the passage of faeces out of the body. The internal sphincter forms the terminal fibres of the GI tract. Under conscious, voluntary control, the external sphincter is continuous with the puborectalis muscle. Between the two is a narrow, fatty intersphincteric space. Differences in pelvic anatomy and body habitus between the sexes result in variations in morphology and mesorectal fat distribution that influences disease progression and management.

Large area surface coils (Figs I.1 & I.2) provide high detail imaging over a large field of view. Despite this, the use of an intracavity coil may be preferred when greater detail is required regarding proximal disease (Fig I.17). Note that coils designed for intracavity examination are specifically designed for the anatomy of interest and are not interchangeable. Using an endorectal coil for anal imaging will most likely result in the coil sitting too superiorly, the anus being outside the field of view.

# Imaging planes: Routine sequences

## Position:

- Supine, head first or feet first
- Arms should be kept above the imaging coil, either resting on the upper chest or above the head.

## Other considerations:

- Removing or using only a low pillow under the head may help the patient feel less encumbered and, depending on the bore length, allow them to see out of the bore.
- Administration of an anti-spasmodic just before imaging will alleviate peristalsis that can degrade image quality.

## Sagittal

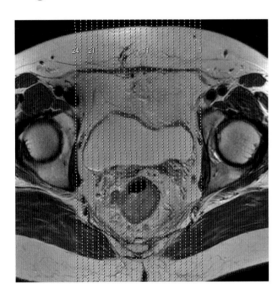

Figure 4.2 Sagittal planned on an axial image. (North Shore Radiology)

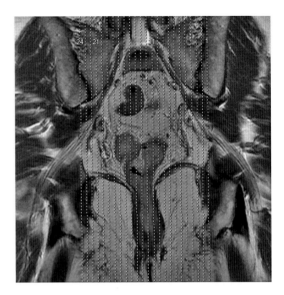

Figure 4.3 Sagittal planned on a coronal image. (North Shore Radiology)

## Alignment:

- True sagittal.

## Coverage:

*Superior to inferior:*
- L5/S1 intervertebral space to anal verge (Fig 4.4)

*Lateral to medial:*
- Pelvic brim on each side

*Posterior to anterior:*
- Sacrum to symphysis pubis.

## Demonstrates:

- Anatomy of the rectum/anus and location of a suspected mass
- Sacral destruction by metastatic extension
- Tumour spread to structures anterior to the rectum.

# Axial

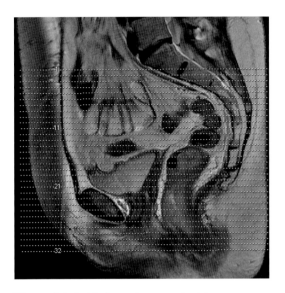

**Figure 4.4** Axial planned on a sagittal image.
(North Shore Radiology)

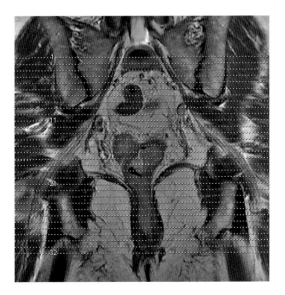

**Figure 4.5** Axial planned on a coronal image.
(North Shore Radiology)

## Alignment:

• True axial.

## Coverage:

*Superior to inferior:*
• First sacral segment to anal verge

*Lateral to medial:*
• Pelvic brim on each side

*Posterior to anterior:*
• Sacrum to symphysis pubis.

## Demonstrates:

• Survey extent of any mass within the rectum
• Parametrial invasion and lymph node extension
• Sacral destruction by metastatic extension
• Mesorectal fat and fascia, assisting in surgical planning
• Permits volumetric analysis of mesorectal compartment.

# Coronal

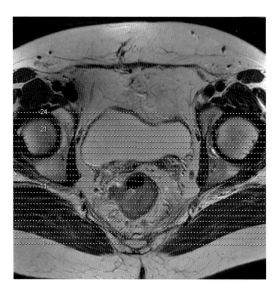

Figure 4.6  Coronal planned on an axial image.
(North Shore Radiology)

## Alignment:

- True coronal.

## Coverage:

- As for sagittal plane.

## Demonstrates:

- Breech of the levator ani in tumour extension
- Differentiation of supra/infralevator abscess:
    - medial displacement with infralevator abscess
    - lateral displacement with supralevator abscess.

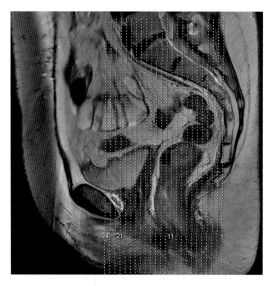

Figure 4.7  Coronal planned on a sagittal image.
(North Shore Radiology)

# Short axis (axial) oblique, rectum

These images are intended to provide higher spatial resolution than the true axial scans.

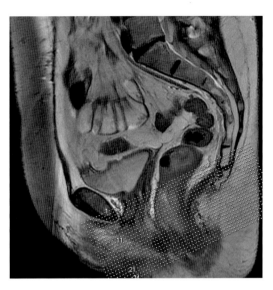

Figure 4.9 Axial oblique planned for a lesion located on a flexure to demonstrate the inferior portion of the rectum and involvement of the anus. (North Shore Radiology)

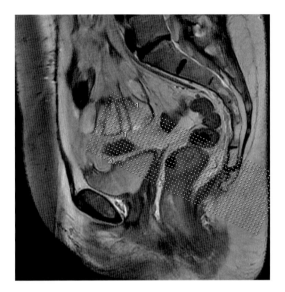

Figure 4.8 Axial oblique planned for a lesion located on a flexure to demonstrate the superior portion of the rectum. (North Shore Radiology)

## Alignment:

- Perpendicular to the long axis of the rectal canal at the level of a mass
- More than one set of data and angles may be required to adequately demonstrate pathology, particularly on a flexure.

## Coverage:

- As required for the mass. Ensure at least one extra slice above and below the mass so it is covered completely.

## Demonstrates:

- Radial disease extension, used to determine the potential tumour-free circumferential resectable margin.

# Short axis (axial) oblique, anus

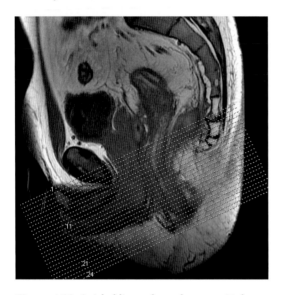

Figure 4.10 Axial oblique planned on a sagittal image for the anorectal junction.
(North Shore Radiology)

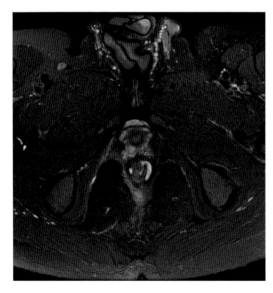

Figure 4.11 Two fistulae, one originating at 1 o'clock and wrapping to the left, the other present at 9 o'clock.
(North Shore Radiology)

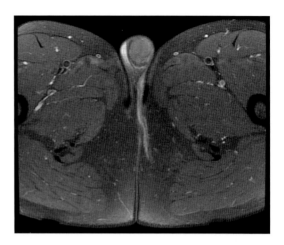

Figure 4.12 Fistula extension to the left scrotum.
(North Shore Radiology)

## Alignment:

- Perpendicular to the long axis of the anal canal
- These images mimic the surgeon's view when the patient is in the lithotomy position.

## Coverage:

*Superior to inferior:*
- Women: distal rectum to anal verge
- Men: distal rectum to testes

*Lateral to medial:*
- Ischial spines on each side

*Posterior to anterior:*
- Coccyx to symphysis pubis:
  - in men, be sure there is no tract extending into the testes (Fig 4.12).

## Demonstrates:

- Involvement of anal sphincters in tumour spread
- Number, radial origin and direction of anal fistula tract(s)
- Extensions coming off fistulae
- Extent of fistula permeation through the pelvis
- Fistula classification, according to the level of origin and sphincter involvement.

## Imaging planes: Supplementary sequences

# Long axis (coronal) oblique, anus

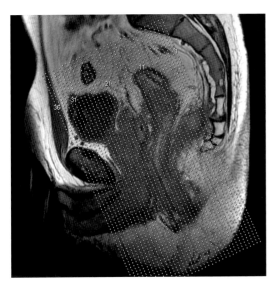

Figure 4.13  Coronal oblique anus planned on a sagittal image.
(North Shore Radiology)

## Alignment:

- Parallel to the long axis of the anal canal.

## Coverage:

- As for short axis plane of anal canal.

## Demonstrates:

- Involvement of anal sphincters with low-lying tumours
- Number, radial origin and direction of anal fistulae tract(s)
- Extensions coming off fistulae
- Extent of fistula permeation through the pelvis
- Fistula classification according to the level of origin and sphincter involvement.

# Chapter 4.2  Female pelvis

## Indications:

- Endometriosis
- Metastasis
- Cancer of the uterus, cervix or ovaries
- Benign uterine lesions, e.g. leiomyoma (fibroid)

- Vaginal adenomyosis
- Pelvic floor dysfunction (PFD)
- Vesicovaginal or rectovaginal fistulae.

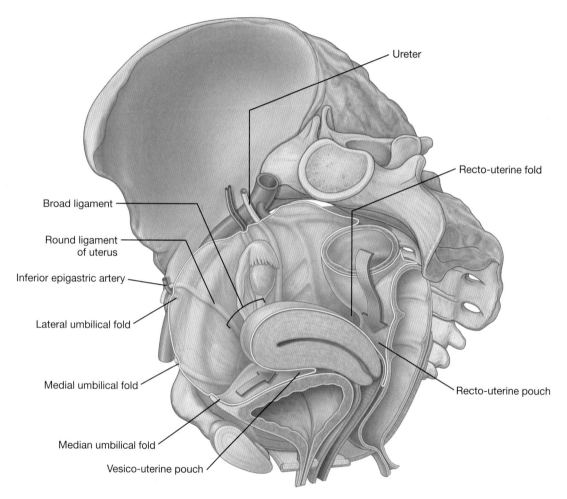

Figure 4.14  Pelvic viscera of the female.
(from Drake, Gray's Anatomy for Students 2e, with permission)

# Coils and patient considerations

Within the middle compartment of the pelvis between the rectum (posterior compartment) and the bladder (anterior compartment), the vagina forms the initial portion of the female reproductive system, joining with the cervix to expand into the uterus. At the uterine fundus on each side, the fallopian tubes deliver ova from the ovaries. Separated from the peritoneal cavity by the broad and round ligaments, the uterus moves to accommodate the degree of bladder or bowel filling.

Beginning caudally at the perineum, the vulva surrounds the vagina which extends cranially to meet the cervix. Angled posteriorly, the transition between the two is marked by an interposing of fibres that creates the anterior and posterior fornices. The transition is also marked by a change in angle as the cervix tips anteriorly, leaning the uterus toward the bladder.

From cervix to apex, the uterus is a long multi-layered muscular structure. Centrally, the highly vascular endometrium is shed on a regular basis during menstruation in the reproductive years. Beneath this the muscular myometrium forms the bulk of the tissue, divided into two zones. Peripherally, the uterus is contained within the perimetrium. Finally, the peritoneum overlies the superoposterior uterus. The anteverted uterus described is the most common, but occasionally a retroverted position may be encountered. Imaging planes must be adjusted accordingly.

The pelvic sling comprises three layers. The muscular levator ani forms the intermediate layer. Superiorly, the endopelvic fascia is a continuation of the peritoneum and connective tissue, while caudally, the urogenital diaphragm is mostly formed by connective tissue and the deep transverse muscle. Poor function of the sling through trauma or surgery leads to relaxation with or without organ prolapse. Imaging for PFD examines this sling and its effectiveness in supporting all three pelvic compartments. In contrast to the other indications, it involves imaging at both rest and during valsalva. Measurements are made from the static and dynamic images to quantify pelvic floor incompetence and determine conservative or surgical management.

An imaging coil with a large field of view is necessary for complete inspection of pelvic disease (Figs I.1 & I.2). However, for detailed imaging of the cervix or vagina, a dedicated intra-cavity coil may provide greater detail of local disease. As mentioned earlier, coils designed for intra-cavity examinations are not interchangeable; a coil designed specifically for the area of interest is required.

# Imaging planes: Routine sequences

## Position:

- Supine, head or feet first
- Keep arms above the pelvis if possible. If not, rest by the sides.

## Other considerations:

- Administration of an anti-spasmodic just before imaging will alleviate peristalsis that can degrade image quality.
- For examination of PFD:
  - ask the patient to void both the bowels and bladder prior to imaging to limit the possibility of incontinence
  - place absorbent padding beneath the buttocks and ensure that leakage into the scanner is prevented with plastic barriers
  - underpants, pessaries and incontinence pads must be removed
  - keep the legs separated enough to permit the degree of organ prolapse to be assessed.

## Sagittal

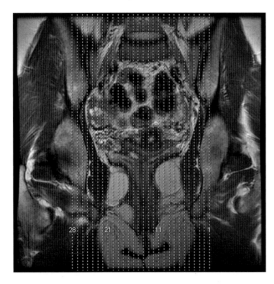

**Figure 4.15** Sagittal planned on a coronal image. (North Shore Radiology)

## Alignment:

- True sagittal.

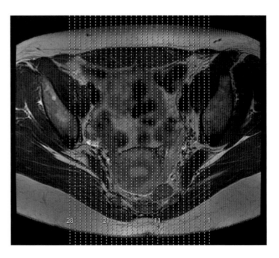

**Figure 4.16** Sagittal planned on an axial iamge. (North Shore Radiology)

## Coverage:

*Superior to inferior:*
- Lumbosacral junction to vulva
- Extend coverage if prolapse goes more caudally

*Lateral to medial:*
- Most indications: true pelvis
- PFD: targeted to the midline only, to show prolapse through the compartmental hiatuses

*Posterior to anterior:*
- Sacrococcygeal spine to symphysis pubis.

## Demonstrates:

- Anteroposterior angulation of reproductive organs, for planning oblique planes
- Zonal anatomy of the uterus (on T2 weighted imaging)
- Location of masses within the vagina or uterus
- Impingement of masses on the bladder or bowel
- Vesicovaginal or rectovaginal fistulae
- Pouch of Douglas
- Pelvic diaphragm and relative displacement on valsalva.

# Axial

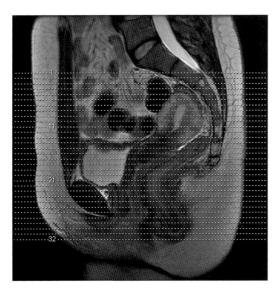

Figure 4.17 Axial planned on a sagittal image.
(North Shore Radiology)

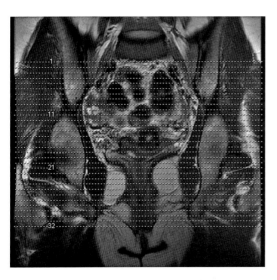

Figure 4.18 Axial planned on a coronal image.
(North Shore Radiology)

## Alignment:

· True axial.

## Coverage:

*Superior to inferior:*
· Fundus of uterus to inferior aspect of the vagina or prolapsed organs, whichever is lower
· Severe PFD may result in multi-organ prolapse. Ensure complete coverage of pelvic contents.

*Lateral to medial:*
· True pelvis

*Posterior to anterior:*
· Sacrum to symphysis pubis.

## Demonstrates:

· Survey of pelvic contents both above and below the levator ani
· Endometriosis within the pelvis, between bowel loops, bladder and reproductive organs
· Parametrial spread and lymph node involvement of malignant disease
· Vesicovaginal or rectovaginal fistulae
· Pelvic diaphragm and organ prolapse
· Levator ani symmetry.

# Coronal

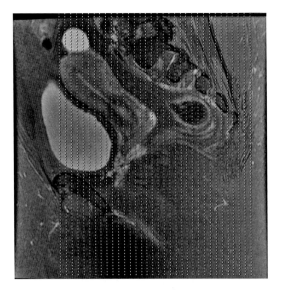

Figure 4.19 Coronal planned on a sagittal image.
(North Shore Radiology)

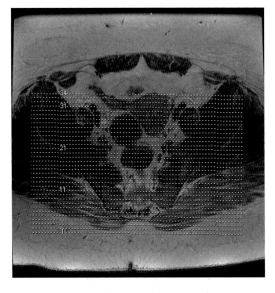

Figure 4.20 Coronal planned on an axial image.
(North Shore Radiology)

## Alignment:

- True coronal.

## Coverage:

*Superior to inferior:*
- Lumbosacral junction to inferior aspect of the vagina

*Lateral to medial:*
- True pelvis

*Posterior to anterior:*
- Sacrum to uterine fundus (or cervix if the uterus is retroverted).

## Demonstrates:

- Integrity of the vaginal fornices, disruption of which increases suspicion of tumour aggression.
- Involvement of pelvic sidewalls with large tumours and compromise of the pelvic sling.
- Ureteric obstruction due to a large mass.

# Axial oblique

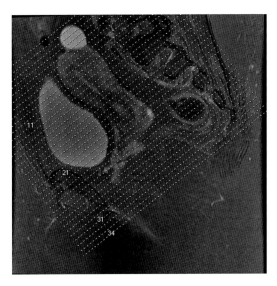

Figure 4.21 Axial oblique uterus planned on a sagittal image. Note the increased coverage to include the cyst superior to the fundus.
(North Shore Radiology)

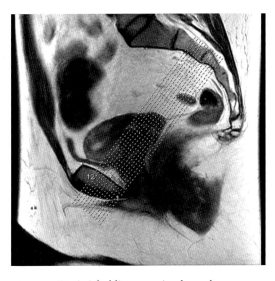

Figure 4.22 Axial oblique cervix planned on a sagittal image.
(North Shore Radiology)

## Alignment:

- Perpendicular to the long axis of the uterus (Fig 4.21), cervix (Fig 4.22) or vagina, as clinical indications require.

## Coverage:

*Superior to inferior:*
- Uterus: fundus of uterus to cervicovaginal junction
- Cervix: vaginal fornices to uterine isthmus
- Vagina: cervix to perineum
- In all cases, if a mass is present, coverage should be extended to include the lesion.

*Lateral to medial:*
- True pelvis

*Posterior to anterior:*
- Sacrum to urinary bladder.

## Demonstrates:

- Zonal anatomy of uterus and cervix (on T2 weighted images) or of the vagina.
- Depth of malignant extension, assisting with determining disease severity and treatment options.

# Chapter 4.3  Male pelvis

## Indications:

- Palpable mass on digital examination
- Prostate cancer for staging or radiotherapy/ surgical workup
- Cancer
- Prostate and peri-prostatic cysts.

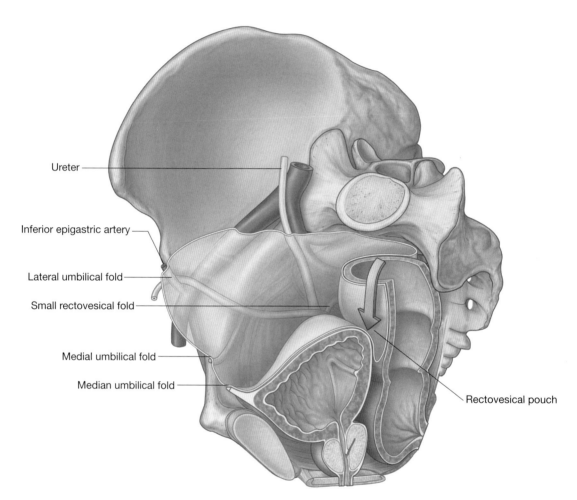

Figure 4.23  Pelvic viscera of the male.
(from Drake, Gray's Anatomy for Students 2e, with permission)

# Coils and patient considerations

Sandwiched between the urogenital diaphragm and the bladder, lesions of the prostate comprise the most common indication for imaging of the male pelvis, often prior to surgical or radiotherapy planning. Sitting deep and low in the pelvis below the symphysis, the prostate encircles the proximal urethra with enlargement of this gland impacting on effective voiding.

The prostate is intimately associated with the inferior surface of the bladder. The gland narrows in a conical fashion to an apex around the urethra, which passes anteriorly within the prostate. The normal prostate usually weighs no more than 8 g, with dimensions of roughly 4 cm near the bladder, 2 cm in anteroposterior length and 3 cm craniocaudally. Immediately posterior to the prostate lies the distal rectum. It is divided into three zones: peripheral, central and transitional, with the outermost layer being fibromuscular tissue.

Superior to the prostate and posterior to the bladder wall, the seminal vesicles merge with the vas deferens carrying sperm from the testes through the ejaculatory duct. These pass through the posterior prostate before anastomosing with the urethra. From bladder to tip of the penis may be up to 20 cm.

Prostate cancer is highly prevalent in men aged over fifty years. MRI may help determine disease aggressiveness. Imaging should include the seminal vesicles to exclude tumour extension. Cystic lesions of the seminal vesicles or remnant müllerian ducts are often incidental findings on MRI or another examinations.

Imaging of the prostate may be performed with a large area surface coil (Figs I.1 & I.2), but greater detail is achieved using an intracavity coil (Fig I.17).

# Imaging planes: Routine sequences

## Position:

- Supine, head or feet first
- Keep arms above the pelvis if possible. If not, rest by the sides.

## Other considerations:

- Patients should be asked to refrain from ejaculation for three days prior to imaging to ensure optimal distension of the seminal vesicles.
- For radiotherapy planning, bladder filling will be a consideration. Check whether an empty or full bladder is required for your particular treatment facility.
- Administration of an anti-spasmodic just before imaging will alleviate peristalsis that can degrade image quality.

## Sagittal

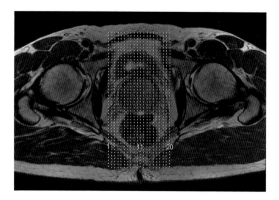

Figure 4.24  Sagittal planned on an axial iamge. (North Shore Radiology)

## Alignment:

- True sagittal.

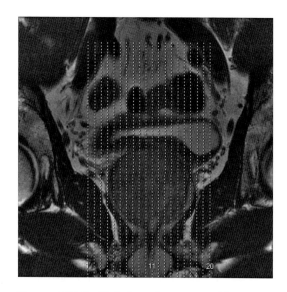

Figure 4.25  Sagittal planned on a coronal image. (North Shore Radiology)

## Coverage:

*Superior to inferior:*
- Superior aspect of the bladder to inferior aspect of the symphysis pubis

*Lateral to medial:*
- True pelvis

*Posterior to anterior:*
- Sacrococcygeal spine to symphysis pubis.

## Demonstrates:

- Prostatic hyperplasia, indenting the urinary bladder
- Defect of the inferior bladder wall after transurethral resection of prostate, possibly mimicking a cyst
- Seminal vesicles
- Extracapsular extension of cancer into the bladder
- Utricle cysts.

# Axial

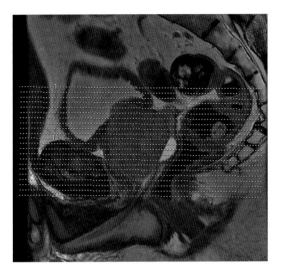

Figure 4.26  Axial planned on a sagittal image.
(North Shore Radiology)

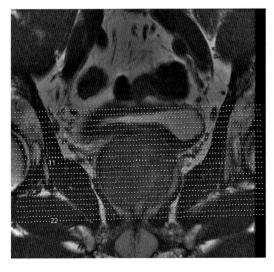

Figure 4.27  Axial planned on a coronal image.
(North Shore Radiology)

## Alignment:

- True axial.

## Coverage:

*Superior to inferior:*
- Seminal vesicles to inferior aspect of the prostate

*Lateral to medial:*
- True pelvis

*Posterior to anterior:*
- Sacrococcygeal spine to symphysis pubis.

## Demonstrates:

- Extracapsular extension of disease, particularly into the retrovesicular space
- Cystic degeneration of benign prostatic hyperplasia (BPH) in the transitional zone
- Seminal vesicles and vas deferens.

# Coronal

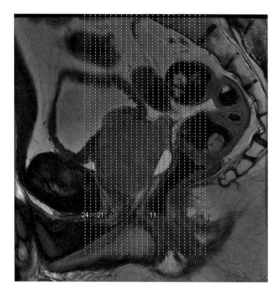

**Figure 4.28** Sagittal planned on a coronal image.
(North Shore Radiology)

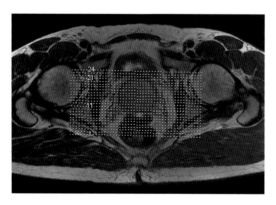

**Figure 4.29** Sagittal planned on an axial image.
(North Shore Radiology)

## Alignment:

- True coronal.

## Coverage:

*Superior to inferior:*
- Superior aspect of the bladder to inferior aspect of the symphysis pubis

*Lateral to medial:*
- True pelvis

*Posterior to anterior:*
- Retrovesicular space to anterior wall of the prostate.

## Demonstrates:

- BPH and cystic degeneration in the transitional zone
- Extracapsular extension of cancer superiorly and laterally into the bladder and levator ani
- Seminal vesicles.

# Chapter 4.4  Testes

## Indications:

- Further evaluation of testicular mass after ultrasound, e.g. testicular carcinoma, seminoma, metastasis, epidermoid cyst, testicular lymphoma.
- Undescended testes or confirmation of testicular agenesis.
- Clarification of intra- versus extra-testicular mass, if not verified by ultrasound.

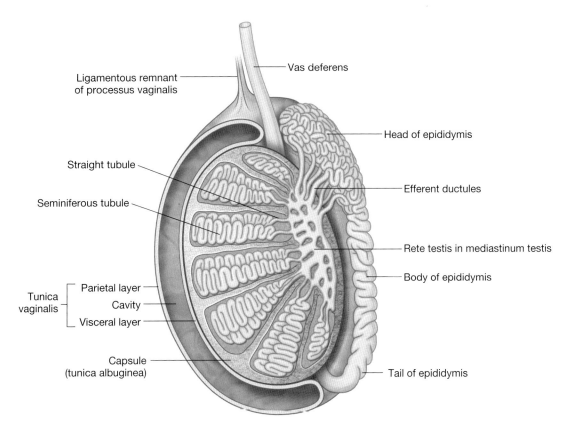

Figure 4.30  Section through one testis.
(from Drake, Gray's Anatomy for Students 2e, with permission)

## Coils and patient considerations

Outside the pelvic cavity, the testes are contained within the tunica albuginea. Divided by septa, the seminiferous tubules radiate around the head of the epididymis. The tubules converge to form tubuli recti, then merge again forming rete testis, before draining into the efferent tubules at the testicular hilum. Piercing the tunica albuginea, these efferent tubules become the head of the epididymis. The individual tubules continue to merge until a single tube is left, at which point it becomes known as the vas deferens. The vas deferens enters the pelvis via the inguinal canal along with the testicular arteries and veins, nerves and lymphatic vessels as the spermatic cord.

Although MRI is generally used in an adjunctive role to ultrasound, it can prove useful in determining the exact location of a lesion and its spread. Malignancy can invade the epididymis and spread to the pelvic lymph nodes. Although CT would be the modality of choice in the evaluation of lymphatic spread, imaging of the pelvis at MRI with a large field of view coil may be requested. A smaller imaging coil is preferred for imaging of the testes in isolation to permit greater image detail. A pair of large dual coils similar to those in Figure I.16 could be an appropriate choice.

# Imaging planes: Routine sequences

## Position:

- Supine, head or feet first
- Keep arms above the pelvis.

## Other considerations:

- Place a towel beneath the testes to raise them ensuring that they are level, and position the penis lying over the lower abdomen to one side out of the area of interest.
- A second, warmed towel laid over the genitals will keep the coil from lying directly on the skin and prevent the scrotum from contracting due to cold.

## Axial

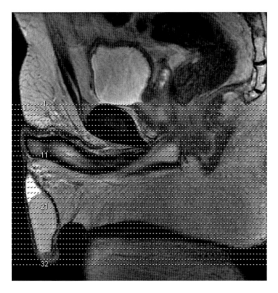

Figure 4.31 Axial planned on a sagittal image.
(North Shore Radiology)

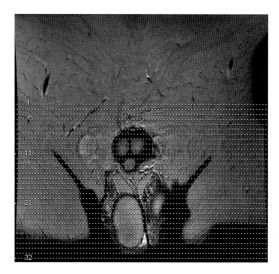

Figure 4.32 Axial planned on a coronal image.
(North Shore Radiology)

## Alignment:

- True axial.

## Coverage:

*Superior to inferior:*
- Superior aspect of the symphysis pubis to inferior aspect of the tunica vaginalis

*Lateral to medial:*
- Inguinal canal on each side

*Posterior to anterior:*
- Symphysis pubis to anterior testicular surface

## Demonstrates:

- Extension of malignancy to epididymis and spermatic cord
- Testicular hilum and the radial septations within the testes
- Undescended testes within the inguinal canal
- Vas deferens.

# Coronal

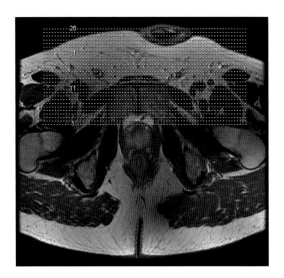

Figure 4.33  Coronal planned on an axial image.
(North Shore Radiology)

## Alignment:

· True coronal.

## Coverage:

· As for axial.

## Demonstrates:

· Undescended testes, sitting above or within
  the inguinal canal
· Epididymis and spermatic cord.

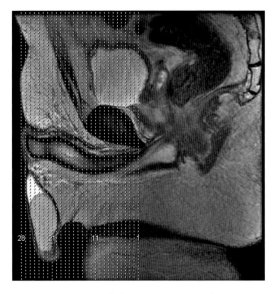

Figure 4.34  Coronal planned on a sagittal image.
(North Shore Radiology)

# Imaging planes: Supplementary sequences

## Sagittal

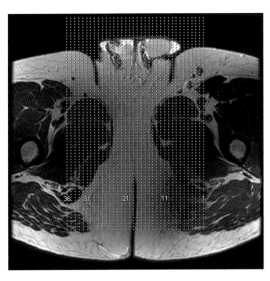

Figure 4.35 Sagittal planned on an axial image.
(North Shore Radiology)

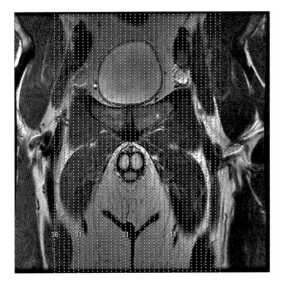

Figure 4.36 Sagittal planned on a coronal image.
(North Shore Radiology)

## Alignment:

- True sagittal.

## Coverage:

- As for axial.

## Demonstrates:

- Spermatic cord entering the inguinal canal.

# Chapter 4.5  Fetal brain

## Indications:

- Clarification of ultrasound findings, e.g. absent corpus callosum, large or asymmetric ventricles, posterior fossa abnormality.
- Fetal viability, particularly in twin pregnancies where one has a demonstrated abnormality.

## Coils and patient considerations

While imaging for any gross fetal anomaly may be requested, a common indication is to confirm concerns about cerebral development. This is the region focused on in this section.

There is significant variation between the stages of fetal development and the corresponding imaging appearances. MR imaging acts as an effective adjunct in the confirmation of equivocal ultrasound results, and will often form part of the workup prior to genetic counselling in cases of suspected congenital abnormalities.

Expecting a fetus to cease moving during a scan is often little more than a dream. Successfully imaging the unborn child without maternal sedation may be a matter of re-adjusting imaging planes and frequently repeating sequences until a series of rapid fire images with no motion artefact have been acquired. Each scan should be planned from the most recently completed datasets, so that changes in fetal position are accommodated. The degree of coverage for the fetal brain is similar to that used for a routine brain examination.

# Imaging planes: Routine sequences

## Position:

- Supine, head or feet first
- Keep arms above the pelvis.

## Other considerations

- Fasting for four hours prior to the examination alleviates peristalsis that may degrade image quality. Use of an anti-spasmodic is not favoured in pregnancy.
- If the pregnancy is at an advanced stage, the mother may be unable to lie flat without becoming lightheaded. Rolling the patient a little to one side will alter the weight distribution.
- Sedation of the fetus can be achieved by sedating the mother, reducing problems with motion artifacts. This is not always used.

## Axial uterus

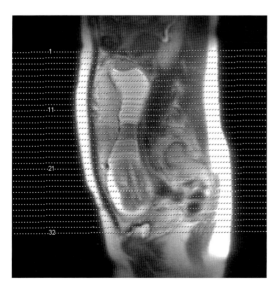

Figure 4.37  Axial uterus planned on a sagittal image.
(North Shore Radiology)

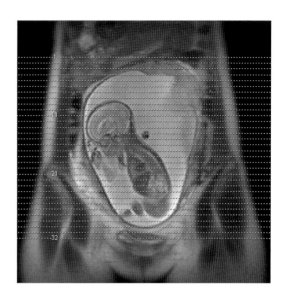

Figure 4.38  Axial uterus planned on a coronal image.
(North Shore Radiology)

## Alignment:

- True axial.

## Coverage:

*Superior to inferior:*
- Uterine fundus to symphysis pubis

*Lateral to medial:*
- Abdominal wall on each side

*Posterior to anterior:*
- Spine to anterior abdominal wall.

## Demonstrates:

- Orientation of the fetus enabling planning of the first clinical image
- Overview of placental morphology.

# Sagittal

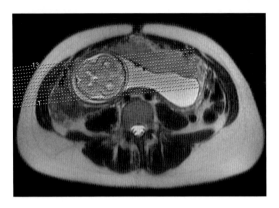

Figure 4.39 Sagittal fetal brain planned on an axial image.
(North Shore Radiology)

## Alignment:

· Parallel to the falx.

## Coverage:

*Inferior to superior:*
· Foramen magnum to vertex

*Lateral to medial:*
· Parietal lobes on each side

*Posterior to anterior:*
· Occipital to frontal lobes.

## Demonstrates:

· Appropriate development of the corpus callosum
· Posterior fossa development, especially the vermis.

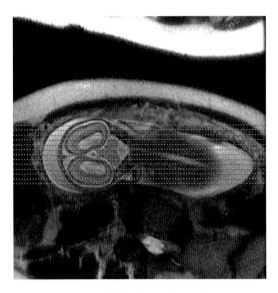

Figure 4.40 Sagittal fetal brain planned on a coronal image.
(North Shore Radiology)

# Axial

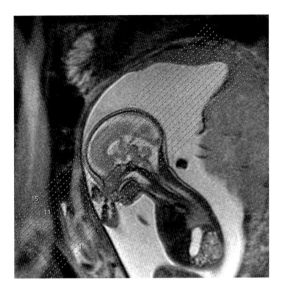

Figure 4.41 Axial fetal brain planned on a sagittal image.
(North Shore Radiology)

## Alignment:

- Parallel to a line joining the splenium and genu of the corpus callosum and perpendicular to the falx.
- If there is agenesis of the corpus callosum, parallel to the floor of the frontal lobe.

## Coverage:

- As for sagittal.

## Demonstrates:

- Ventricular size and symmetry
- Parenchymal development or damage
- Sulcal development, used to assess maturation of the brain.

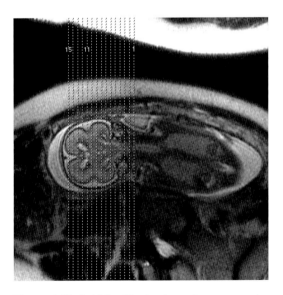

Figure 4.42 Axial fetal brain planned on a coronal image.
(North Shore Radiology)

# Coronal

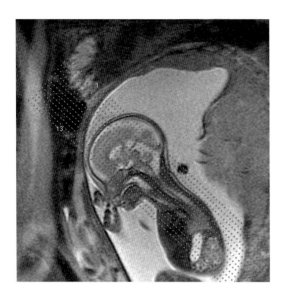

Figure 4.43 Coronal fetal brain planned on a sagittal image.
(North Shore Radiology)

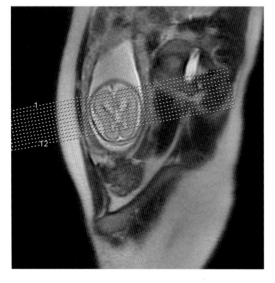

Figure 4.44 Coronal fetal brain planned on an axial image.
(North Shore Radiology)

## Alignment:

· Perpendicular to the brainstem and falx.

## Coverage:

· As for axial.

## Demonstrates:

· Appropriate development of the corpus callosum
· Parenchymal development or damage
· Sulcal development.

# Chapter 4.6  Pelvic arteries

## Indications:

- Renal transplant compromise
- Vascular claudication
- Stenosis
- Thrombosis
- Congenital anomalies or malformations, e.g. arteriovenous malformation.

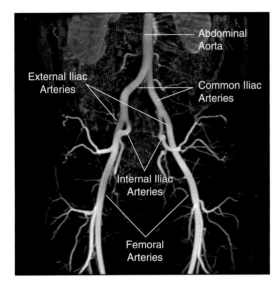

Figure 4.45  MIP image of the pelvis, demonstrating the arterial supply.
(Midland MRI)

## Coils and patient considerations

The abdominal aorta lies slightly to the left of midline anterior to the spine, bifurcating into the left and right common iliac arteries at the level of the fourth lumbar vertebra. These short segments of vessel further divide into the internal and external iliac arteries at the level of the intervertebral disc between the fifth lumbar vertebra and the first sacral segment. The organs, viscera and muscles of the pelvis and medial thigh are fed by the internal iliac artery, further dividing into anterior and posterior divisions deeper in the pelvis, each giving off several branches.

The external iliac artery courses medial to the psoas major muscle, before being renamed the femoral artery after passing beneath the inguinal ligament to enter the thigh. The point of entry to the thigh lies midway between the anterior superior iliac spine (ASIS) and the symphysis pubis, just above the femoral head.

A large area surface coil is required (Figs I.1 & I.2). Plans in this section assume the use of a gadolinium-based contrast medium.

# Imaging planes: Routine sequences

## Position:

- Supine, head or feet first
- Keep arms above the pelvis or overhead if possible. If not, rest by the sides.

## Other considerations:

- The legs should be separated and relaxed. A small pad beneath the knees may alleviate back pain.

## Coronal

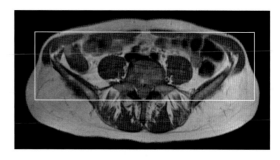

**Figure 4.47** Coronal volume planned on an axial image.
(North Shore Radiology)

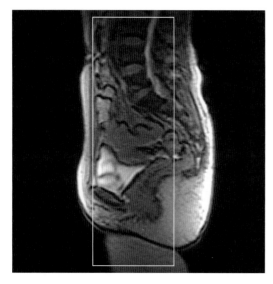

**Figure 4.46** Coronal volume planned on a sagittal image.
(North Shore Radiology)

## Alignment:

- Parallel to the long axis of the distal aorta and proximal iliac arteries.
- Planning using a good quality axial 2D dataset on which cross-sections of the major vessels can be seen may assist in ensuring adequate coverage.

## Coverage:

*Superior to inferior:*
- Third lumbar vertebra to lesser trochanters

*Lateral to medial:*
- Greater trochanters on each side

*Posterior to anterior:*
- Sacrococcygeal spine to mid thigh.

## Demonstrates:

- Stenosis
- Dissection
- Data should be post-processed as MIPs.

# Further reading

Allen SD, Gada V, Blunt DM 2007 Variation of mesorectal volume with abdominal fat volume in patients with rectal carcinoma: assessment with MRI. British Journal of Radiology 80(952):242–247

Amin RS, Nikolaidis P, Kawashima A et al 1999 Normal anatomy of the fetus at MR imaging. Radiographics 19:S201–S214

Baumgartner BR, Bernardino ME 1989 MR Imaging of the cervix: off-axis scan to improve visualization of the zonal anatomy. American Journal of Roentgenology 153(5):1001–1002

Bloch BN, Lenkinski RE, Rofsky NM 2008 The role of magnetic resonance imaging (MRI) in prostate cancer imaging and staging at 1.5 and 3 tesla: The Beth Deaconess Medical Center (BIDMC) approach. Cancer Biomark 4(4): 251–262

Boyadzhyan L, Raman SS, Raz S 2008 Role of static and dynamic MR imaging in surgical pelvic floor dysfunction. Radiographics 28(4):949–967

Coakley FV, Glenn OA, Qayyum A et al 2004 Fetal MRI: A developing technique for the developing patient. American Journal of Roentgenology 184(1):243

Curran S, Akin O, Agildere AM et al 2007 Endorectal MRI of prostatic and periprostatic cystic lesions and their mimics. American Journal of Roentgenology 188(5):1373–1379

Halligan S et al 2006 Imaging of fistula in ano. Radiology 239(1):18–33

Hoeffel CC, Aziz L, Mourra N et al 2006 MRI of rectal disorders. American Journal of Roentgenology 187(3):W275–284

Hricak H, Williams RD, Spring DB et al 1983 Anatomy and pathology of the male pelvis by magnetic resonance imaging. American Journal of Roentgenology 141(6):1101–1110

Klessen C, Rogalla P, Taupitz M 2007 Local staging of rectal cancer: the current role of MRI. European Radiology 17(2):379–389

Kim B, Kawashima A, Ryu JA et al 2008 Imaging of the seminal vesicle and vas deferens. Radiographics 29(4):1105–1121

Kim W, Rosen MA, Langer JE et al 2007 US-MR imaging correlation in pathologic conditions of the scrotum. Radiographics 27(5):1239–1253

Limperopoulos C, Robertson RL, Khwaja OS et al 2008 How accurately does current fetal imaging identify posterior fossa anomalies. American Journal of Roentgenology 190:1637–1643

Loubeyre P, Petignat P, Jacob S et al 2009 Anatomic distribution of posterior deeply infiltrating endometriosis and MRI after vaginal and rectal gel opacification. American Journal of Roentgenology 192(6):1625–1631

Parikh JH, Barton DP, Ind TE et al 2008 MR imaging features of vaginal malignancies. Radiographics 28(1):49–63

Sella T, Schwartz LH, Swindle PW et al 2004 Suspected local recurrence after radical prostatectomy: endorectal coil MR imaging. Radiology 231(2):379–385

Stark DD, Bradley WG 1999 Magnetic Resonance Imaging, Vol. I, 3rd edn, Mosby, St Louis, pp 635–651

Suzuki C, Torkzad MR, Tanaka S et al 2008 The importance of rectal cancer MRI protocols on interpretation accuracy. World Journal of Surgical Oncology 6:89. Online. Available: http://www.ncbi.nlm.nih.gov/pmc/articles/PMC2533319/pdf/1477-7819-6-89.pdf, 14 Mar 2011

Woodward PJ, Sohaey R, O'Donoghue MJ et al 2002 From the Archives of the AFIP: Tumors and tumor-like lesions of the testis: Radiologic-pathologic correlation. Radiographics 22(1):189–216

# Section 5

# Upper limb

# Chapter 5.1  Shoulder

## Indications:

- Rotator cuff tear
- Assessment of supraspinatous retraction and fatty infiltration, with a view to surgical repair
- Glenohumeral instability and associated labral lesions:
  - Bankart/Pethes (anterior instability) +/− Hills-Sachs lesion
  - Reverse Bankart (posterior instability) +/− reverse Hills-Sachs lesion

  - Superior labral anterior posterior (SLAP)
  - Anterior labroligamentous periosteal sleeve avulsion (ALPSA)
  - Humeral avulsion glenoid ligament (HAGL)
- Bicipital tendonitis
- Osteonecrosis.

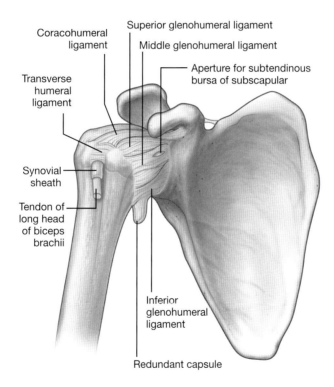

Figure 5.1 Capsule of the glenohumeral joint.
(From Drake, Gray's Anatomy for Students 2e, with permission)

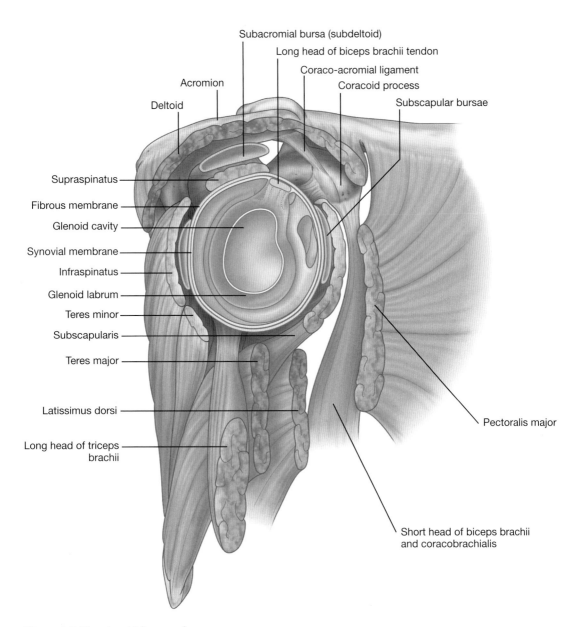

Figure 5.2 The glenoid fossa en face.
(from Drake, Gray's Anatomy for Students 2e, with permission)

## Coils and patient considerations

Examinations of the shoulder generally focus on the glenohumeral joint and the supporting structures. The shallow glenoid fossa is deepened by a ring of labral cartilage, to which attach the various ligaments and tendons. Injuries to the labrum result in instability, inducing pain and functional disruption. Causes may be either traumatic as with dislocation, or degenerative.

The rotator cuff is the major stabiliser of the shoulder, formed by the supraspinatous, infraspinatous, teres minor and subscapularis tendons. Damage to the supraspinatous tendon (SST) is common with age-related damage, acromial spurs and trauma making this a very frequent cause of shoulder dysfunction. Patients with partial or complete tears of the SST are generally unable to raise the arm above the head.

There is some variation in the design of imaging coils for this body region (see Figs I.14–I.16 for examples). Coils with independent posterior and anterior elements (Fig I.16) need to be carefully aligned to ensure adequate signal and minimise respiratory motion, as the anterior element may move. Moulded, rigid designs (Figs I.14 & I.15) do not suffer this problem, although heavy respiration may still impact on image quality due to movement of the anterior chest wall.

With all cases, respiratory motion is reduced by keeping the chest from coming into contact with the anterior aspect of the coil. It is often advantageous to rotate the patient to the side of interest as a means of minimising contact. However, it may not be possible to completely prevent contact with more heavyset patients. Pads and velcro straps should be employed when positioning the patient to stabilise the coil and arms before commencing scanning, but take care that any velcro bands are not affected by patient breathing. All patients should be instructed to breathe normally during image acquisition, but requested not to take deeper breaths. When speaking to patients between series give them the opportunity to take a few deep breaths before continuing.

# Imaging planes: Routine sequences

## Position:

- Supine obliqued slightly to the side of interest, generally head first. This will assist in bringing the shoulder closer to isocentre, improving image quality.
- Upper arm parallel to the table. This may require some padding to be placed under the elbow to correct any posterior tilt distally.
- Arm by side, hand externally rotated 5°–20° to extend and separate the supraspinatous tendon from the infraspinatous on the axial and coronal views. Rotation also better demonstrates the anterior labrum–ligament complex, often injured in anterior dislocations.

## Other considerations:

- Patients with rotator cuff injuries often suffer significant and worsening shoulder pain when supine. Sufficient support under the head and neck are essential.
- If rotating the hand externally exacerbates the pain, then it is better to leave it in a neutral position. Less commonly, patients cannot tolerate even this position so allow them to place the hand on the lower pelvis provided there is no skin-to-skin contact (use sponges to separate). Laxity in the supraspinatous tendon may limit the conspicuity of tears, but it may be necessary if image blurring due to patient motion is to be prevented.

## Axial

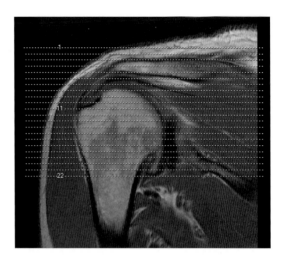

Figure 5.3 Axial planning on a coronal image. (North Shore Radiology)

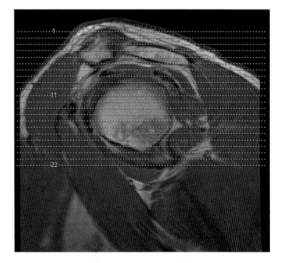

Figure 5.4 Axial planning on a sagittal image. (North Shore Radiology)

## Alignment:

- Usually true axial
- If the humeral head is sitting in an abnormally high position, some angulation to the supraspinatous muscle may be required.

## Coverage:

*Superior to inferior:*
- Acromion to inferior glenoid rim

*Lateral to medial:*
- Deltoid to supraspinatous fossa

*Posterior to anterior:*
- Anterior to posterior skin surfaces.

## Demonstrates:

- Supraspinatous tendon retraction
- Anterior (Bankart) or posterior (reverse Bankart, Hills-Sachs) labral and humeral head damage
- Rotator cuff tears
- Biceps tendon displacement
- Cystic changes in the humeral head due to impingement.

## Sagittal

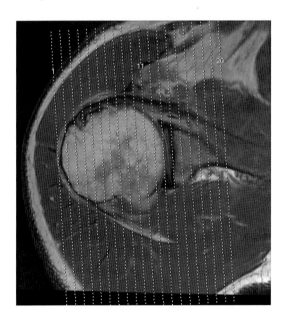

Figure 5.5 Sagittal planning on an axial image. (North Shore Radiology)

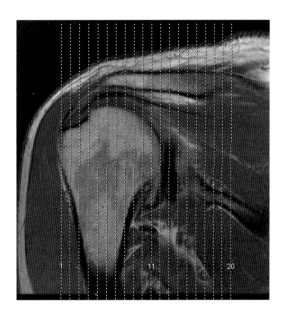

Figure 5.6 Sagittal planning on an coronal image. (North Shore Radiology)

## Alignment:

- Parallel to glenoid surface.

## Coverage:

*Superior to inferior:*
- Acromion to inferior glenohumeral joint

*Lateral to medial:*
- Greater tuberosity to supraspinatous fossa

*Posterior to anterior:*
- Anterior to posterior skin surfaces.

## Demonstrates:

- Supraspinatous muscle retraction, atrophy and fatty infiltration.
- Tendon or muscle hyperintensity, indicative of injury. This is easier to appreciate without the competing signal of fat that may be present in chronically injured joints.
- Bankart and reverse Bankart lesions.

# Coronal

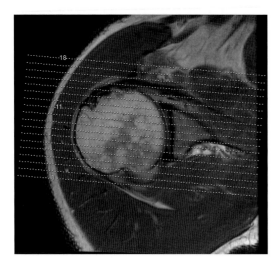

Figure 5.7 Coronal planning on an axial image.
(North Shore Radiology)

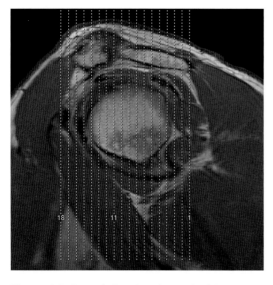

Figure 5.8 Coronal planning on a sagittal image.
(North Shore Radiology)

## Alignment:

- In plane with the supraspinatous tendon at its insertion (Fig 5.9).
- Incorrect angulation (Figs 5.10 & 5.11) may result in foreshortening of the supraspinatous tendon, affecting demonstration of tendon tears.
- The supraspinatous tendon may have retracted with a complete tear and not be visible. In this case scans may be planned to the blade of the scapula (Fig 5.11).

## Coverage:

*Superior to inferior:*
- Acromion to inferior glenoid labrum

*Lateral to medial:*
- Greater tuberosity to supraspinatous fossa

*Posterior to anterior:*
- Infraspinatus to pectoralis major muscles.

## Demonstrates:

- Irregularity of the rotator cuff, partial or full thickness supraspinatous tendon tear
- Biceps tendon insertion
- Hills-Sachs deformity posterosuperiorly
- Superior (SLAP) lesion
- Inferior glenohumeral ligament damage (HAGL)
- Relationship between the supraspinatous and acromio-clavicular joint.

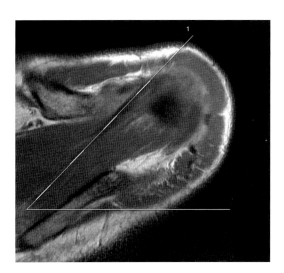

Figure 5.9  Correct coronal alignment, along the supraspinatous tendon.
(North Shore Radiology)

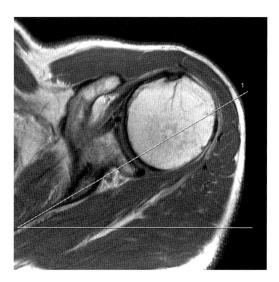

Figure 5.11  Incorrect alignment to the blade of the scapula.
(North Shore Radiology)

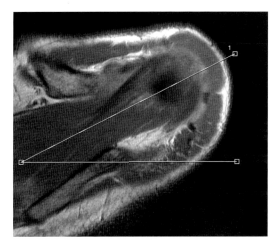

Figure 5.10  Incorrect alignment to the muscle belly.
(North Shore Radiology)

# Imaging planes: Supplementary sequences

## ABER (abduction external rotation)

### Position:

- Supine, head first.
- Arm abducted and externally rotated, resting above the head, palm facing the roof of the bore (Fig 5.12). This is designed to release stress on the anterior labrum, making a detachment more easily demonstrated. Be sure to keep the hand separated from the head.
- Patient may lie completely supine for this view.

### Other considerations:

- Not all patients will be capable of attaining this position.
- It may be ill-advised to attempt this position in patients being examined for recurrent dislocations.
- For patients unable to do ABER, an ADIR may be an alternative position (see below).

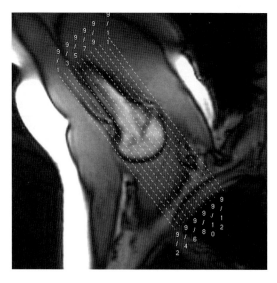

Figure 5.13  ABER planning on a coronal image. (North Shore Radiology)

### Alignment:

- Shaft of humerus on a coronal localiser

### Coverage:

*Superior to inferior:*
- Acromion to inferior glenoid labrum

*Lateral to medial:*
- Humeral head to supraspinatous fossa

*Posterior to anterior:*
- Infraspinatus to pectoralis major muscles.

### Demonstrates:

- Impingement of the infraspinatous tendon by the posterosuperior glenoid
- Anterior band of the inferior glenohumeral ligament
- Lamination of supraspinatous tears posteriorly
- Differentiation of Perthes lesions (undisplaced Bankart) from complete avulsion (Bankart).

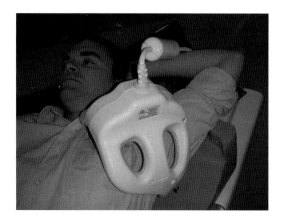

Figure 5.12  ABER position. (North Shore Radiology)

# ADIR (ADduction internal rotation)

## Position:

- Supine, head first.
- Arm adducted and internally rotated so that the palm rests pronated on the table underneath the lower back, increasing pressure on the posterior aspect of the joint, resulting in distension of the anterior capsule (Fig 5.14).
- Suggested only for MR arthrography, when the joint capsule is sufficiently distended by contrast.
- Place thermally protective padding between the body and the bore to minimise the risk of burns.

## Other considerations:

- Patients being examined for anterior instability should be positioned with care, so as to not inadvertently dislocate the humeral head.

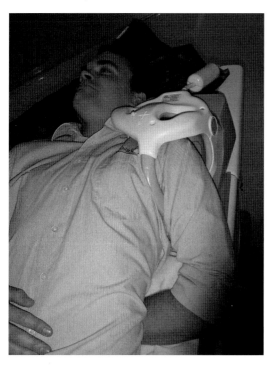

Figure 5.14 ADIR position.
(North Shore Radiology)

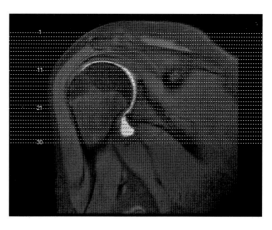

Figure 5.15 ADIR planning an axial image.
(North Shore Radiology)

## Alignment:

- True axial.

## Coverage:

*Superior to inferior:*
- Acromioclavicular joint to inferior labrum

*Lateral to medial:*
- Humeral head to glenoid

*Posterior to anterior:*
- Posterior to anterior skin surfaces.

## Demonstrates:

- Classification of labral lesions, specifically Bankart, Perthes or ALPSA.

# Chapter 5.2  Elbow

## Indications:

- Epicondylitis
  - Golfer's elbow (medial epicondylitis)
  - Tennis elbow (lateral epicondylitis)
- Biceps tendon tear
- Osteochondral lesions

- Instability
- Loose bodies
- Neuropathies
- Tumour
- Trauma.

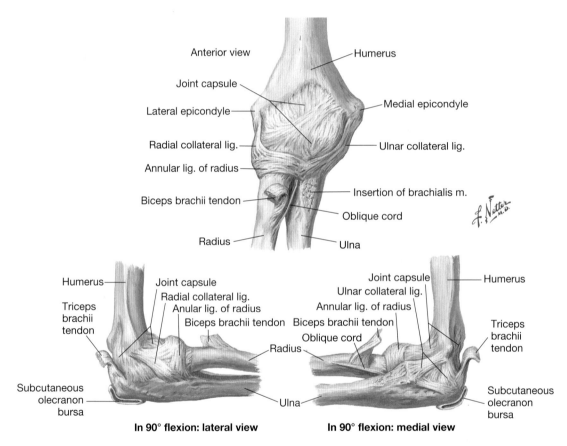

**Figure 5.16** Ligaments of the elbow.
(Netter illustration from www.netterimages.com ©Elsevier Inc. All rights reserved.)

## Coils and patient considerations

The radial head articulates with the capitellum of the humerus proximally. Just below the head, a flatter medial surface articulates with the ulnar, while the distal biceps tendon attaches to the radial tuberosity. The proximal ulna pivots between the epicondyles and the trochlea and capitellum, the olecranon sliding into a fossa posteriorly in extension and the coronoid similarly received into its own fossa anteriorly in flexion.

The ulnar and radial collateral ligaments support the joint, in conjunction with the annular ligament. A synovial membrane with invaginations that accommodate a broad range of movements encapsulates the joint.

A number of muscles surround the elbow joint, divided into anterior, posterior, medial and lateral compartments. Certain muscles in the medial and lateral compartments merge to form the common flexor and extensor tendons, respectively. It is these tendons that become inflamed with epicondylitis. Injuries involving the distal biceps tendon are uncommon, but when requiring examination this tendon benefits from particular attention with a dedicated view (Ch 5.2 Supplementary sequences).

Positioning the patient with the arm by the side is preferred, and may be best tolerated but is not always practical due to limitations of body habitus and field homogeneity. The greatest field homogeneity is located at the centre of the scanner; hence a prone 'Superman' type position may be preferred. A pillow under the axillae and upper chest reduces the degree of extension required at the shoulder. Extra support in the axilla using pads further helps with stabilisation.

Ideally the palm should be supinated, but in many cases the patient experiences pain so pronation may be the only option. Supination of the palm may be better tolerated when the patient is supine.

A range of imaging coils is available to examine this body region: they are either tubular in design or flexible (for examples, see Figs I.7, I.8, I.11 & I.16). The more cumbersome coils are suitable for use when the patient is positioned with the arm raised above the head, lying prone, while a flexible coil is suitable for imaging with the arm by the side or in fixed flexion.

# Imaging planes: Routine sequences

## Preferred position:

- Supine, generally head first.
- Arm by side, palm supinated. This causes the radius to rotate away from the ulna and extends the lateral collateral ligament.
- Ensure the patient is moved to the non-symptomatic side, enabling the elbow of interest to be as close as possible to the middle of the scanner.
- If the patient is touching the bore on the opposite side, place thermally protective padding between the two to minimise the risk of burns.

## Alternative position:

- Prone, arm of interest extended over the head with the palm supinated.
  - If the 'Superman' position is employed, the ulnar collateral ligament will not be sufficiently extended making demonstration of subluxation difficult to assess.

## Axial

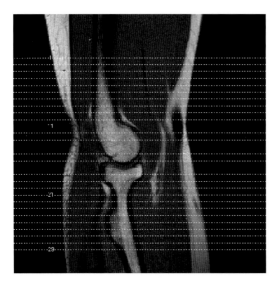

Figure 5.17  Axial planning on a sagittal image.
(North Shore Radiology)

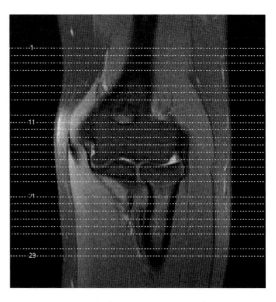

Figure 5.18  Axial planning on a coronal image.
(North Shore Radiology)

## Alignment:

- Axial to the long axis of the humerus.

## Coverage:

*Superior to inferior:*
- Distal third of humerus to radial tuberosity

*Lateral to medial:*
- Lateral and medial epicondyles

*Posterior to anterior:*
- Skin surfaces.

## Demonstrates:

- Intra-articular loose bodies
- Radial and ulnar collateral ligament insertions
- Distal biceps tendon
- Nerves.

# Coronal

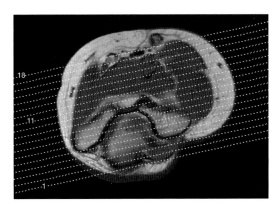

Figure 5.19 Coronal planning on an axial image.
(North Shore Radiology)

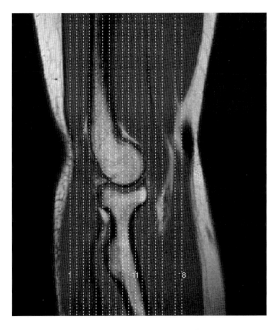

Figure 5.20 Coronal planning on a sagittal image.
(North Shore Radiology)

## Alignment:

- Parallel to a line bisecting the medial and lateral epicondyles.

## Coverage:

*Superior to inferior:*
- Distal third of humerus to radial tuberosity

*Lateral to medial:*
- Lateral to medial epicondyles

*Posterior to anterior:*
- Olecranon to biceps muscle belly.

## Demonstrates:

- Radial and ulnar collateral ligaments
- Attachments of the common extensor and flexor tendons
- Articular surfaces and radial head.

# Sagittal

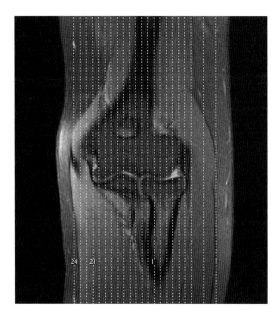

**Figure 5.21** Sagittal planning on a coronal image.
(North Shore Radiology)

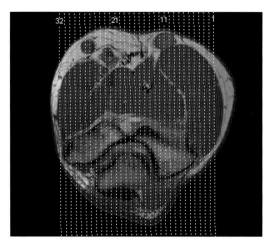

**Figure 5.22** Sagittal planning on an axial image.
(North Shore Radiology)

## Alignment:

· Perpendicular to a line bisecting the medial and lateral epicondyles.

## Coverage:

*Superior to inferior:*
· Distal third of humerus to radial tuberosity

*Lateral to medial:*
· Medial and lateral collateral ligament insertions

*Posterior to anterior:*
· Olecranon to biceps muscle belly.

## Demonstrates:

· Intra-articular loose bodies
· Radial head and capitellar injuries
· Secondary assessment of the radial and ulnar collateral ligaments
· Triceps tendon
· Posterior subluxation of the radial head due to posterolateral instability.

## Imaging planes: Supplementary sequences

### FABS (flexion abduction in supination)—coronal biceps tendon

#### Position:

- Prone, head first
- Humerus abducted 180° over the head with the elbow bent to 90°, thumb supinated, i.e. aligned superiorly facing the ceiling (Fig 5.23).

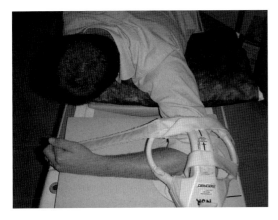

**Figure 5.23** FABS position.
(North Shore Radiology)

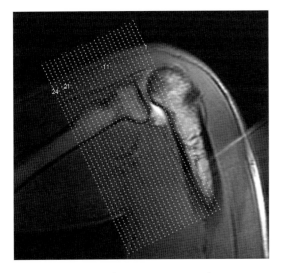

**Figure 5.24** FABS planning on a sagittal image.
(North Shore Radiology)

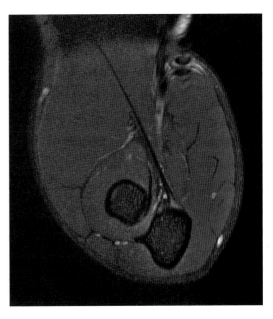

**Figure 5.25** FABS image, showing the biceps tendon.
(North Shore Radiology)

### Alignment:

- Parallel to the distal biceps tendon as seen on a sagittal view of the joint
- If the tendon is not visible, plan nearly perpendicular to the shaft of the radius.

### Coverage:

*Superior to inferior:*
- Distal third of humerus to olecranon

*Lateral to medial:*
- Skin edge on each side

*Posterior to anterior:*
- Humeral shaft to radial tuberosity
- Be sure to cover the entire tuberosity as the attachment broadens, with fibres also attaching to the ulna.

### Demonstrates:

- Distal biceps tendon integrity along its length, without bowing
- This is the best plane for differentiating between partial and complete tendon tears.

# Chapter 5.3 Wrist

## Indications:

- Triangular fibrocartilage complex injury (TFCC)
- Kienbock's disease (lunate osteonecrosis)
- Scaphoid injury, fracture, non-union +/− osteonecrosis
- Scapholunate (SL) disruption
- Arthritis (RA, OA)
- Distal radio-ulnar joint disruption (DRUJ)
- Tumour, e.g. pigmented villonodular synovitis (PVNS)
- De Quervain's or stenosing tenosynovitis (washerwoman's sprain)
- Tendinopathy
- Instability
- Ganglion.

## Coils and patient considerations

The complex wrist joint, comprising the bones of the carpus, the distal radioulnar joint (DRUJ) and the carpometacarpal joints, forms a significant portion of musculoskeletal injuries. Falls on the outstretched hand may damage the radioulnar joint or the scaphoid, with other carpals less frequently injured. Stress-related injuries are common in athletes who load or compress the joint repeatedly, as with gymnasts.

Beginning medially the proximal row of carpals consists of the pisiform, triquetrum, lunate and scaphoid. The distal row includes the hamate, capitate, trapezoid and trapezium. Each of the carpals and the long bones are interconnected by multiple ligaments, while muscles are found in the forearm, acting via the tendinous attachments that extend or flex the wrist. The extensor tendons are the extensor carpi radialis brevis, extensor carpi radialis longus, extensor carpi ulnaris, extensor digitorum communis and extensor pollicis longus. The flexor tendons are the flexor carpi radialis, flexor carpi ulnaris, flexor digitorum superficialis and flexor pollicis longus.

The ulnar and radial collateral ligaments, classed as extrinsic ligaments, extend from the bones of the same names and attach to the triquetrum and pisiform medially and the scaphoid laterally. Ligaments interconnecting carpal bones (but not the pisiform, considered a sesamoid) are described as intrinsic.

Radiofrequency coils with a small field of view provide the best spatial resolution for the small structures of the wrist (Figs 1.10 & 1.12). If a patient presents in a back-slab or plaster, it is worth asking the referrer if it may be removed before scanning. This will enable the smallest possible coil to be used.

As with the elbow, the patient may be positioned supine with the arm by the side or prone with the arm extended over the head. The latter places the wrist in the most homogeneous area of the magnet.

Kinematic imaging of the wrist uses a non-ferromagnetic device to move the joint through incremental degrees of radial/ulnar deviation, imaging in the coronal plane. These may be viewed as stills or in a cine fashion. Likewise, sagittal images may be taken with the wrist in extended, neutral and flexed positions.

## Ligaments of wrist

**Posterior (dorsal) view**

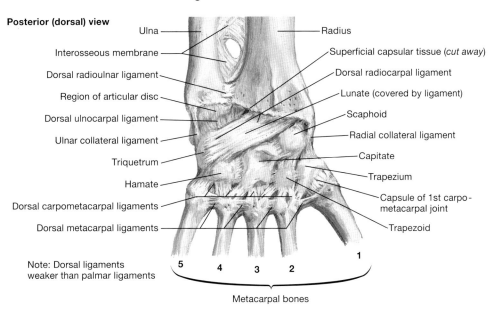

Ulna — 
Interosseous membrane — 
Dorsal radioulnar ligament — 
Region of articular disc — 
Dorsal ulnocarpal ligament — 
Ulnar collateral ligament — 
Triquetrum — 
Hamate — 
Dorsal carpometacarpal ligaments — 
Dorsal metacarpal ligaments — 

Radius
Superficial capsular tissue (*cut away*)
Dorsal radiocarpal ligament
Lunate (covered by ligament)
Scaphoid
Radial collateral ligament
Capitate
Trapezium
Capsule of 1st carpo-metacarpal joint
Trapezoid

Note: Dorsal ligaments weaker than palmar ligaments

5   4   3   2   1

Metacarpal bones

**Coronal section: dorsal view**

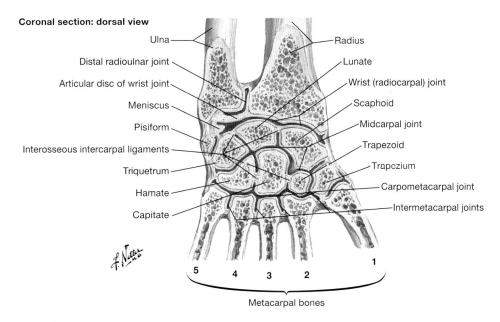

Ulna — 
Distal radioulnar joint — 
Articular disc of wrist joint — 
Meniscus — 
Pisiform — 
Interosseous intercarpal ligaments — 
Triquetrum — 
Hamate — 
Capitate — 

Radius
Lunate
Wrist (radiocarpal) joint
Scaphoid
Midcarpal joint
Trapezoid
Trapezium
Carpometacarpal joint
Intermetacarpal joints

5   4   3   2   1

Metacarpal bones

Figure 5.26 Palmar and volar wrist.

# Imaging planes: Routine sequences

## Preferred position:

- Prone, head first
- Palm pronated in the imaging coil, fingers extended.

## Alternative position:

- Supine, arm by the side with the palm pronated in the coil, fingers extended
- Alternately, the palm may face the hip so that the thumb points to the ceiling.

## Axial

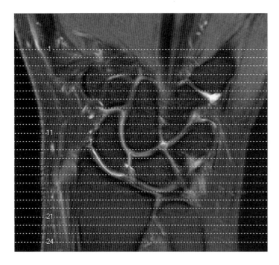

**Figure 5.27** Axial planning on a coronal.
(North Shore Radiology)

## Alignment:

- Axial to the distal radio-ulnar joint.

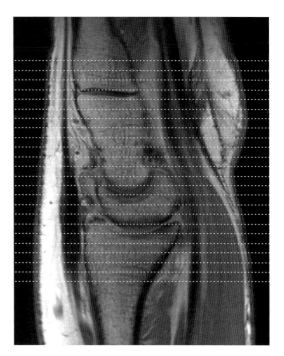

**Figure 5.28** Axial planning on a sagittal image.
(North Shore Radiology)

## Coverage:

*Proximal to distal:*
- DRUJ to metacarpophalangeal joints

*Lateral to medial:*
- First to fifth carpometacarpal joints and including the DRUJ

*Posterior to anterior:*
- Entire carpus and carpal tunnel, from volar to dorsal aspects.

## Demonstrates:

- Carpal tunnel
- Bony attachments of the scapholunate ligament
- Ganglions
- Tendinopathy
- Scapholunate and lunotriquetrum ligaments.

# Coronal

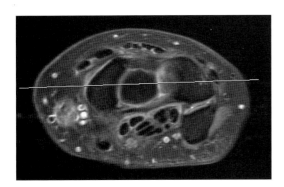

Figure 5.29  Coronal plane.
(North Shore Radiology)

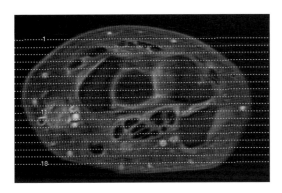

Figure 5.30  Coronal planning on an axial image.
(North Shore Radiology)

## Alignment:

- Parallel to a line bisecting the scaphoid, lunate and pisiform.

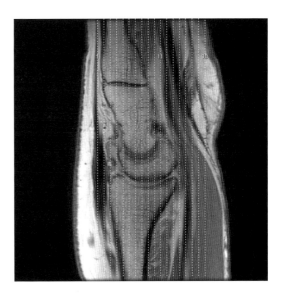

Figure 5.31  Coronal planning on an sagittal image.
(North Shore Radiology)

## Coverage:

*Proximal to distal:*
- DRUJ to metacarpophalangeal joints

*Lateral to medial:*
- First to fifth carpometacarpal joints and including the DRUJ

*Posterior to anterior:*
- Entire carpus and carpal tunnel, from volar to dorsal aspects.

## Demonstrates:

- TFCC
- Central portion of the scapholunate ligament
- Carpal degeneration and alignment
- Intrinsic ligaments.

# Sagittal

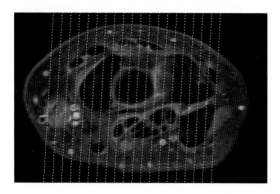

Figure 5.32 Sagittal planning on an axial image.
(North Shore Radiology)

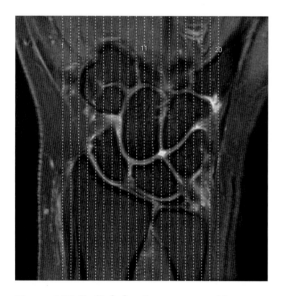

Figure 5.33 Sagittal planning on a coronal image.
(North Shore Radiology)

## Alignment:

- Perpendicular to a line bisecting the scaphoid, lunate and pisiform.

## Coverage:

*Proximal to distal:*
- DRUJ to metacarpophalangeal joints

*Lateral to medial:*
- First to fifth carpometacarpal joints and including the DRUJ

*Posterior to anterior:*
- Dorsal and palmar skin surfaces.

## Demonstrates:

- Radiocarpal and ulnar-carpal alignment
- Carpal degeneration and alignment
- TFCC
- Inflammation of volar or palmar ligaments.

# Chapter 5.4 Thumb and fingers

## Indications:

- Glomus tumour of the nail bed
- Giant cell tendon sheath tumour (also known as PVNS)
- Tendon injury or phalangeal fracture

- Ulnar collateral ligament tear, at the first metacarpophalangeal joint (gamekeeper's or skier's thumb)
- Arthritis (RA, OA).

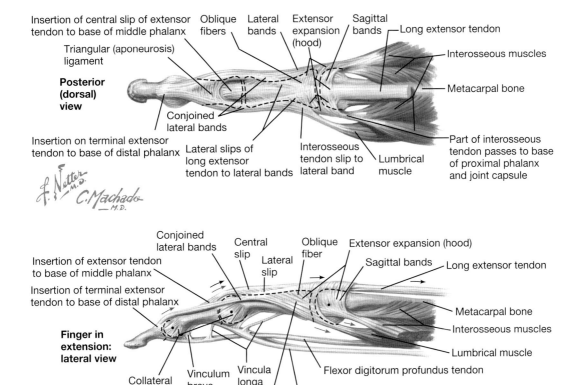

Figure 5.34 Dorsal and sagittal finger.
(Netter illustration from www.netterimages.com ©Elsevier Inc. All rights reserved.)

## Coils and patient considerations

The digits of the hands are subject to many injuries and, sometimes, disease processes.

Aligned at 45° to the rest of the digits of the hand, the thumb requires dedicated and separate alignment for imaging. A moulded wrist coil is generally not suitable for imaging of the fingers as the field of view often does not encompass the distal phalanges. A flexible coil (example in Fig 1.11) or a longer tubular coil is preferred. Paired dual coils (Fig 1.12) also provide good signal with small fields of view, offering high spatial resolution imaging of the small phalanges and joints of the hand and feet.

# Imaging planes: Routine sequences

## Preferred position:

- Prone, head first
- Palm pronated in the imaging coil, fingers extended
- If the patient is touching the bore on the opposite side, place thermally protective padding between the two to minimise the risk of burns.

## Alternative position:

- Supine, arm by the side with the palm pronated in the coil, fingers extended
- Alternately, the palm may face the hip so that the thumb points to the ceiling
- A small pad to create space between the body and the hand is useful to assist in preventing phase wrap.

## Axial: thumb

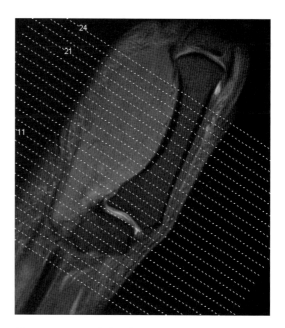

**Figure 5.36** Axial thumb planning on a sagittal image.
(North Shore Radiology)

## Coverage:

*Proximal to distal:*
- Localised joint injury:
    - Proximal to distal midshafts of the phalanges or carpal bones either side of the joint
- Phalanges, tendon diffuse disease:
    - Metacarpophalangel joint to tip of the digit

*Lateral to medial:*
- Lateral to medial skin surfaces

*Posterior to anterior:*
- Skin surfaces.

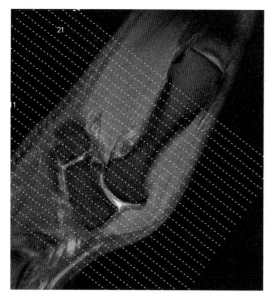

**Figure 5.35** Axial thumb planning on a coronal image.
(North Shore Radiology)

## Alignment:

- Long axis of the finger.

## Demonstrates:

- Flexor and extensor tendon integrity
- Mass lesions
- Joint arthritis.

# Axial: fingers

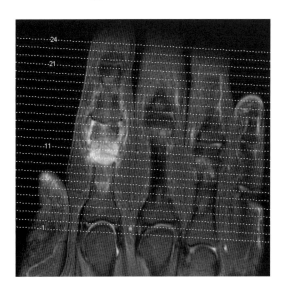

Figure 5.37 Axial planning on a coronal image, aligned to the second digit.
(North Shore Radiology)

## Alignment:

- Long axis of the finger.

## Coverage:

*Proximal to distal:*
- Localised joint injury:
  - Proximal to distal midshafts of the phalanges either side of the joint
- Phalanges, tendon diffuse disease:
  - Metacarpophalangel joint to tip of the digit

*Lateral to medial:*
- Lateral to medial skin surfaces

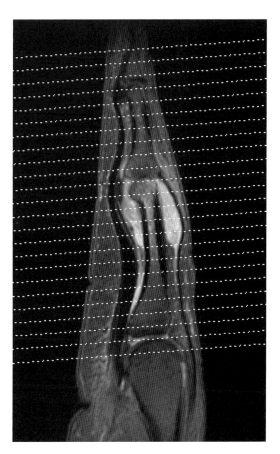

Figure 5.38 Axial planning on a sagittal image, aligned to the second digit.
(North Shore Radiology)

*Posterior to anterior:*
- Skin surfaces.

## Demonstrates:

- Flexor and extensor tendon integrity
- Mass lesions
- Joint arthritis.

# Sagittal

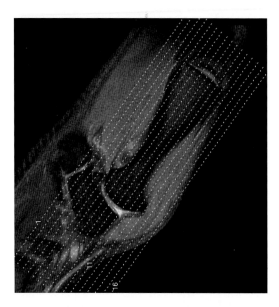

Figure 5.39 Sagittal thumb, focusing on the metacarpal, planned on a coronal image.
(North Shore Radiology)

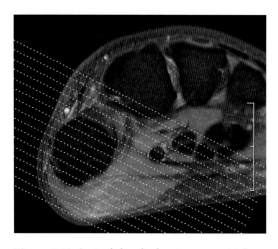

Figure 5.40 Sagittal thumb planning on an axial image.
(North Shore Radiology)

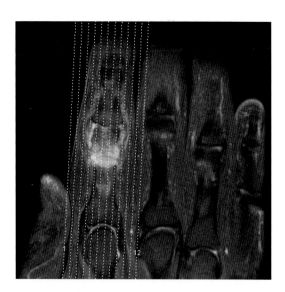

Figure 5.41 Sagittal second digit planned on a coronal image.
(North Shore Radiology)

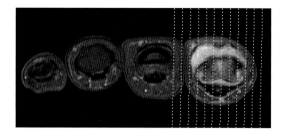

Figure 5.42 Axial second digit planned on a coronal image.
(North Shore Radiology)

## Alignment:

· Shaft of the proximal or distal phalanx of thumb or finger.

## Coverage:

*Proximal to distal:*
· Metacarpophalangeal joint to tip of the digit or metacarpus to metacarpophalangeal joint

*Lateral to medial:*
- One digit either side of that under investigation

*Posterior to anterior:*
- Skin surfaces.

## Demonstrates:

- Flexor tendon integrity
- Joint derangement.

# Coronal

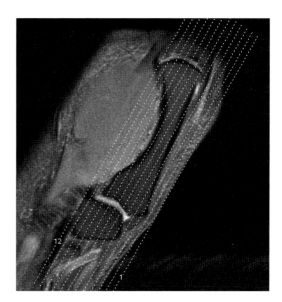

Figure 5.43 Coronal thumb, focusing on the metacarpal, planned on a sagittal image.
(North Shore Radiology)

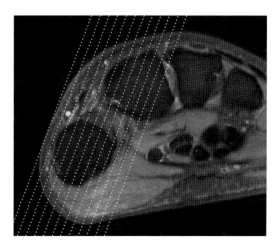

Figure 5.44 Coronal thumb planned on an axial image.
(North Shore Radiology)

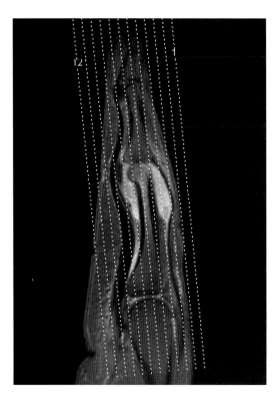

Figure 5.45 Coronal second digit planned on a
sagittal image.
(North Shore Radiology)

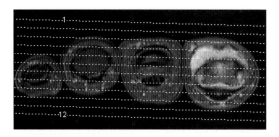

Figure 5.46 Coronal second digit planned on an
axial image.
(North Shore Radiology)

## Alignment:

· Metacarpophalangeal joints.

## Coverage:

*Proximal to distal:*
· Metacarpophalangeal joint to tip of the digit

*Lateral to medial:*
· First to fifth digits

*Posterior to anterior:*
· Skin surfaces.

## Demonstrates:

· Collateral ligament integrity
· Joint derangement.

# Chapter 5.5  Humerus and forearm

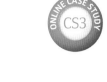

## Indications:

· Tumour or other mass.

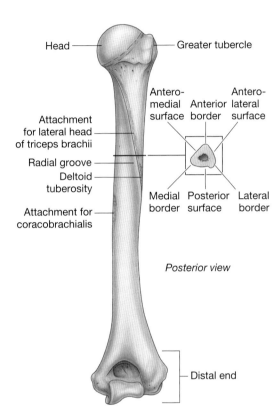

Head — Greater tubercle

Antero-medial surface  Anterior border  Antero-lateral surface

Attachment for lateral head of triceps brachii

Radial groove

Deltoid tuberosity

Medial border  Posterior surface  Lateral border

Attachment for coracobrachialis

*Posterior view*

Distal end

**Figure 5.47** The humerus.
(from Drake, Gray's Anatomy for Students 2e, with permission)

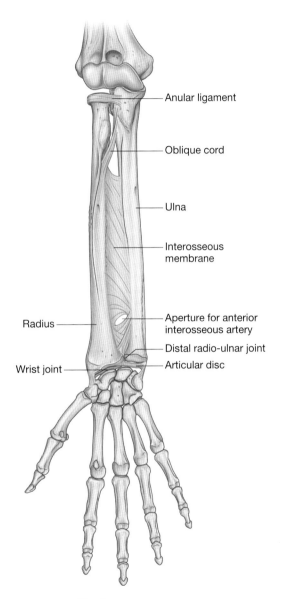

Anular ligament

Oblique cord

Ulna

Interosseous membrane

Radius

Aperture for anterior interosseous artery

Wrist joint

Distal radio-ulnar joint

Articular disc

**Figure 5.48** The forearm.
(from Drake, Gray's Anatomy for Students 2e, with permission)

## Coils and patient considerations

Extending from the glenohumeral joint to the distal radioulnar joint, the long bones of the upper limb require different approaches. Each supported and surrounded by muscles that facilitate abduction and rotation, their proximity to the body provides a challenge in setting up a patient for scanning.

If the patient is fairly mobile, the forearm may be scanned in a tubular coil in a similar manner to the elbow. Alternately, flexible coils (Fig I.11) are often available in a range of sizes for patients who are unable to lie prone with the arm abducted above the head.

For imaging the shaft of the humerus, a large flexible coil may be suitable. In its absence or when a very large field of view is required, a body type coil may be preferred (Figs I.1 & I.2).

In all cases, separation of the limb of interest from the adjacent body is essential to minimise the effects of involuntary patient movement, such as respiration, to prevent aliasing and to minimise the risk of creating conductive loops through the tissues that may result in burns at points of contact.

Scanning long axis images first (coronal or sagittal) enables localisation of pathology and assessment of extent, before planning appropriately targeted axial images.

# Imaging planes: Routine sequences

## Preferred position:

- Prone, head first
- Palm supinated in the imaging coil to unwrap the radius from the ulna, if possible
- Including the joint nearest the region of interest is essential to enable correct orientation of pathology to relevant anatomy.

## Alternative position:

- Supine, arm by the side with the palm supinated in the coil, fingers extended, if possible.

## Coronal

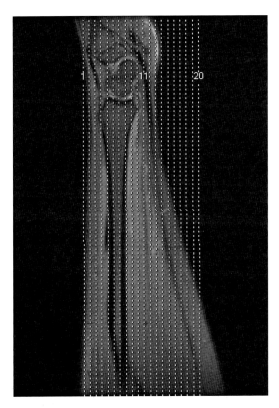

Figure 5.49 Coronal lower arm planned on a sagittal image.
(North Shore Radiology)

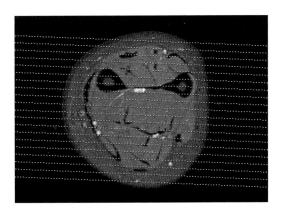

Figure 5.50 Coronal lower arm planned on an axial image.
(North Shore Radiology)

## Alignment:

- For midshaft lesions, align parallel to the interosseous membrane
- If pathology is closer to one joint, align to the joint included for reference
- Localised joint injury:
  - Parallel to the epicondyles at the elbow
  - Parallel to distal radio-ulnar joint at the wrist
  - Align images to the long axis of the bones.

## Coverage:

*Proximal to distal:*
- Wherever possible, both proximal and distal joints should be included
- Include only the joint nearest the region of interest if complete coverage of the bone is not possible

*Lateral to medial:*
- Skin surfaces

*Posterior to anterior:*
- Skin surfaces

## Demonstrates:

- Radial and ulnar shafts
- Cortical integrity.

# Sagittal

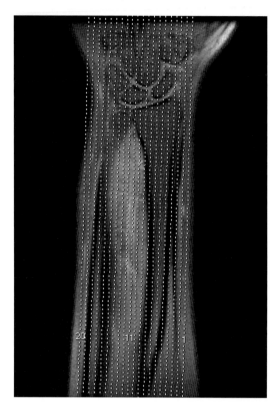

Figure 5.51 Sagittal lower arm planned on a coronal image.
(North Shore Radiology)

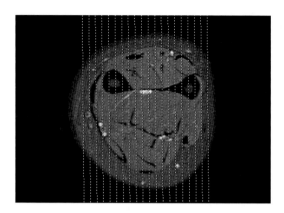

Figure 5.52 Sagittal lower arm planned on an axial image.
(North Shore Radiology)

## Coverage:

*Proximal to distal:*
- Wherever possible, both proximal and distal joints should be included
- Include only the joint nearest the region of interest if complete coverage is not possible

*Lateral to medial:*
- Skin surfaces

*Posterior to anterior:*
- Skin surfaces

## Demonstrates:

- Shafts of the long bones
- Cortical integrity.

## Alignment:

- For midshaft lesions, align perpendicular to the interosseous membrane
- If they are closer to one joint, align to the joint included for reference
- Localised joint injury:
  - Parallel to the epicondyles at the elbow
  - Parallel to distal radio-ulnar joint at the wrist
  - Align images to the long axis of the bones.

# Axial

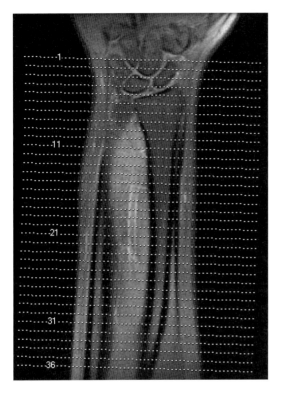

Figure 5.53 Axial lower arm planned on a coronal image.
(North Shore Radiology)

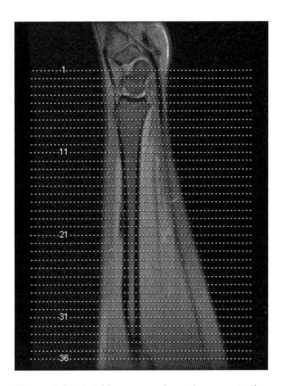

Figure 5.54 Axial lower arm planned on a sagittal image.
(North Shore Radiology)

## Alignment:

- Shafts of the radius and ulna.

## Coverage:

*Proximal to distal:*
- Using the sagittal and/or coronal images, plan slices to cover both proximal and distal to evident pathology
- In the absence of obvious pathology, the entire long bone should be covered

*Lateral to medial:*
- Skin surfaces

*Posterior to anterior:*
- Skin surfaces.

## Demonstrates:

- Shafts of the long bones
- Cortical integrity
- Relationship of neurovascular and musculoskeletal structures.

# Further reading

Carlson CL 2004 The 'J' sign. Radiology 232(3):725–726

Chew ML, Guiffre BM 2005 Disorders of the distal biceps brachii tendon. Radiographics 25(5):1227–1237

Gheno R, Buck FM, Nico MA et al 2010 Differences between radial and ulnar deviation of the wrist in the study of the intrinsic intercarpal ligaments: Magnetic resonance imaging and gross anatomic inspection in cadavers. Skeletal Radiology 39(8):799–805

Giaroli EL, Major NM, Higgins LD 2005 MRI of internal impingement of the shoulder. American Journal of Roentgenology 185(4):925–929

Guiffre BM, Moss MJ 2004 Optimal positioning for MRI of the distal biceps brachii tendon: flexed abducted supinated view. American Journal of Roentgenology 182(4):944–946

Hayter CL, Giuffre BM 2009 Overuse and traumatic injuries of the elbow. Magnetic Resonance Imaging Clinics of North America (17):617–638

Ho-Taek S, Yong-Min H, Sungjin K et al 2006 Anterior–inferior labral lesions of recurrent shoulder dislocation evaluated by MR arthrography in an adduction internal rotation (ADIR) position. Journal of Magnetic Resonance Imaging 23(1):29–35

Khoury V, Cardinal E, Brassard P 2008 Atrophy and fatty infiltration of the supraspinatus muscle: sonography versus MRI. American Journal of Roentgenology 190(4):1105–1111

Lisle DA, Shepherd GJ, Cowderoy GA et al 2009 MR Imaging of traumatic and overuse injuries of the wrist and hand in athletes. Magnetic Resonance Clinics of North America 17:639–654

Ly L, Beall DP, Sanders TG 2003 MR imaging of glenohumeral instability. American Journal of Roentgenology 181(1):203–213

Mackay D, Rangan A, Hide G et al 2003 The objective diagnosis of early tennis elbow by magnetic resonance imaging. Occupational Medicine 53(5):309–312

Passariello R, Mastantuono Mark, Satragno L 2001 Dynamic Magnetic Resonance Imaging of the Hand and Wrist. In: Guglielmi G, van Kuijk C, Genant HK (eds) Fundamentals of Hand and Wrist Imaging. Springer, Berlin, 109–120

Pennekamp W, Gekie C, Nicolas V et al 2006 Abstract: Initial results of shoulder MRI in external rotation after primary shoulder dislocation and after immobilization in external rotation. Fortschritte auf dem Gebiete der Röntgenstrahlen und der Nuklearmedizin 178(4):410–415

Rosenberg ZS, Blutreich SI, Schweitzer ME et al 2008 MRI features of posterior capitellar impaction injuries. American Journal of Roentgenology 190(2):435–441

Tirman PFJ, Bost FW, Steinbach LS et al 1994 MR arthrographic depiction of tears of the rotator cuff: Benefit of abduction and external rotation of the arm. Radiology 192:851–856

Wischer TK, Bredella MA, Genant HK et al 2002 Perthes lesion (a variant of the Bankart lesion): MR imaging and MR arthrographic findings with surgical correlation. American Journal of Roentgenology 178(1):233–237

# Section 6

# Lower limb

# Chapter 6.1 Hip—unilateral

## Indications:

- Enthesopathy or enthesitis, e.g. trochanteric bursitis
- Abductor tendon tear (gluteus minimus or medius that form the rotator cuff of the hip)
- Labral tear

- Arthritis (RA, OA)
- Osteonecrosis (AVN), transient osteoporosis
- Femoro-acetabular impingement (FAI)
- Fracture.

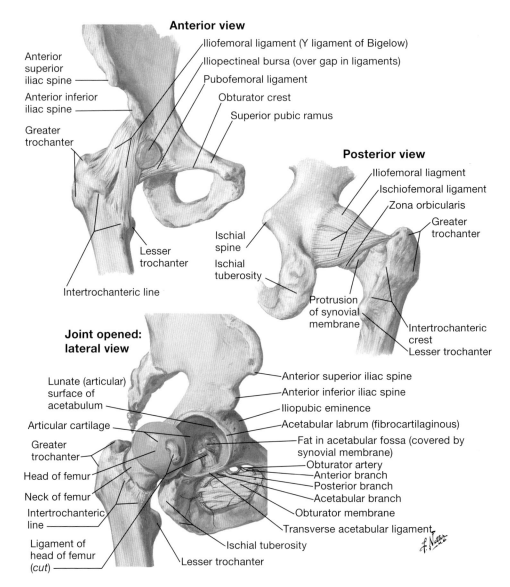

**Anterior view**

Anterior superior iliac spine
Anterior inferior iliac spine
Greater trochanter
Iliofemoral ligament (Y ligament of Bigelow)
Iliopectineal bursa (over gap in ligaments)
Pubofemoral ligament
Obturator crest
Superior pubic ramus
Lesser trochanter
Intertrochanteric line

**Posterior view**

Iliofemoral liagment
Ischiofemoral ligament
Zona orbicularis
Greater trochanter
Ischial spine
Ischial tuberosity
Protrusion of synovial membrane
Intertrochanteric crest
Lesser trochanter

**Joint opened: lateral view**

Lunate (articular) surface of acetabulum
Articular cartilage
Greater trochanter
Head of femur
Neck of femur
Intertrochanteric line
Ligament of head of femur (cut)
Anterior superior iliac spine
Anterior inferior iliac spine
Iliopubic eminence
Acetabular labrum (fibrocartilaginous)
Fat in acetabular fossa (covered by synovial membrane)
Obturator artery
Anterior branch
Posterior branch
Acetabular branch
Obturator membrane
Transverse acetabular ligament
Ischial tuberosity
Lesser trochanter

Figure 6.1 The hip joint.
(Netter illustration from www.netterimages.com ©Elsevier Inc. All rights reserved.)

## Coils and patient considerations

The hip is formed by the articulation of the femoral head with the pelvic acetabulum. The acetabulum is deepened by the cartilaginous labrum forming a 'c' that opens at the acetabular notch to allow passage of the transverse ligament. Ensuring the intimacy and stability of the joint, the articular capsule consists of the iliofemoral, ischiofemoral and pubofemoral ligaments, collectively known as the extracapsular ligaments. Within the joint, the ligamentum teres originates at the acetabular notch, inserting at the fovea of the femur. Damage to the labrum or the supporting ligaments leads to instability.

Imaging of the hip needs to be considered in the context of the suspected underlying pathology and the pelvis as a whole. Consultation with a radiologist to determine whether to image one hip, both hips or the entire pelvis is required, and will alter the protocol and possibly the imaging coil used. A coil with a large field of view (Figs I.1 & I.2) enables imaging of the both hips. A smaller coil may offer better detail for injuries to the labrum (Fig I.16).

Respiratory motion caused by abdominal breathing may induce artefacts when using a large imaging coil. Do not tie the anterior and posterior coil elements too tightly.

The upper limbs should be positioned away from the coil. In most cases simply placing the hands on the chest will suffice, but for patients who are of short stature the arms may need to be raised above the head to prevent the elbows from being within the field when imaging the pelvis. This may also be necessary for larger patients if the elbows cannot comfortably fit within the bore.

# Imaging planes: Routine sequences

## Position:

- Supine, generally feet first.
- Legs straight or at most with a small cushion under the knees to relieve discomfort, with the legs resting in a comfortable neutral position. The feet should be in a similar position so that the head and neck of the femur on each side are imaged in similar positions.
- Arms above the head, away from the imaging coils.

## Other considerations:

- When body habitus causes a large coil to slope downwards towards the legs, sponges can level out the coil preventing it from sliding caudally during the examination. This should also assist in producing consistent signal throughout the images.

## Axial or axial oblique

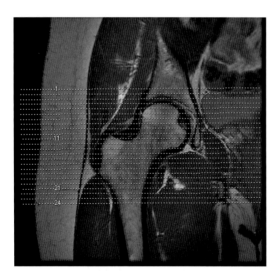

Figure 6.2 Axial planned on a coronal image.
(North Shore Radiology)

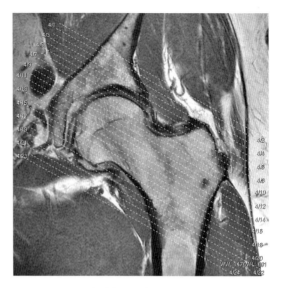

Figure 6.3 Axial oblique planned on a coronal image.
(North Shore Radiology)

## Alignment:

- Axial: for osteonecrosis, transient osteoporosis
  - True transverse orientation
- Axial oblique: for labral or rotator cuff tears (abductor tendons), neck of femur (NOF) fractures and FAI
  - Parallel to the long axis of the neck of femur.

## Coverage:

*Superior to inferior:*
- Axial: superior labrum to lesser trochanter
- Axial oblique: complete coverage of the acetabular labrum

*Lateral to medial:*
- Acetabular rim to trochanteric bursa

*Posterior to anterior:*
- Greater trochanter to anterior acetabular rim, including surrounding musculature.

## Demonstrates:

- Axial oblique:
  - Damage to the anterior or posterior labrum and acetabular cartilage
  - Anteroposterior femoroacetabular alignment
  - Relationship of femoral neck to the acetabulum, particularly when a dysplastic neck results in impingement causing FAI (cam type FAI)
  - Fractures of the neck of the femur.
- Axial:
  - Abductor tendon insertions at the greater trochanter +/− trochanteric bursitis laterally
  - Iiopsoas bursitis anteriorly, possibly indicative of snapping hip syndrome
  - Relationship of the piriformis muscle to the sciatic nerve.

# Coronal or coronal oblique

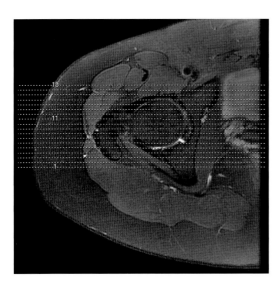

Figure 6.4 Coronal planned on an axial image.
(North Shore Radiology)

## Alignment:

- Coronal: true coronal orientation
- Coronal oblique: parallel to the long axis of the femoral neck.

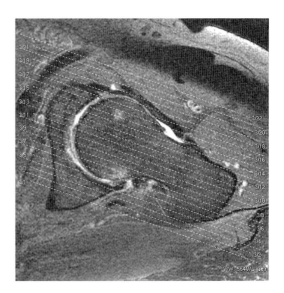

Figure 6.5 Coronal oblique planned on an axial image.
(North Shore Radiology)

## Coverage:

*Superior to inferior:*
- Greater sciatic notch to lesser trochanter

*Lateral to medial:*
- Acetabular rim to trochanteric bursa

*Posterior to anterior:*
- Greater trochanter to anterior acetabulum.

## Demonstrates:

- Acetablular dysplasia
- Superoinferior labral and acetabular damage and sclerosis
- Superoinferior femoro-acetabular alignment
- Lateral labral damage
- Trochanteric bursitis +/− elongation or thickening of the abductor tendons, suggestive of atrophy and/or a tear
- Acetabular and femoral articular cartilage integrity or thinning
- Coronal oblique: alignment and position of the femoral head, particularly important in Perthes' disease.

# Sagittal

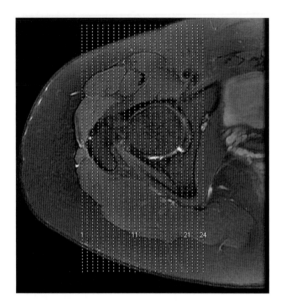

Figure 6.6 Sagittal planned on an axial image.
(North Shore Radiology)

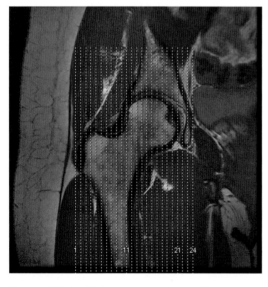

Figure 6.7 Sagittal planned on a coronal image.
(North Shore Radiology)

## Alignment:

- True parasagittal plane or angled 10° medial from the parasagittal plane. Verify with your site.

## Coverage:

*Superior to inferior:*
- Superior acetabulum to lesser trochanter

*Lateral to medial:*
- Acetabular rim to trochanteric bursa

*Posterior to anterior:*
- Greater trochanter to anterior acetabulum and surrounding musculature.

## Demonstrates:

- Damage to the anterosuperior labrum
- Posterior or anterior labral and acetabular damage
- Abductor attachments at the great trochanter
- Femoral head damage associated with osteonecrosis.

# Imaging planes: Supplementary sequences

## Axial: bilateral
### Position:

- As per routine hip sequences.

### Other considerations:

- Nil.

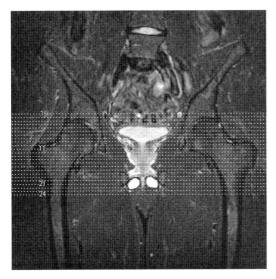

**Figure 6.8** Bilateral hips, axial planned on a coronal image.
(North Shore Radiology)

### Alignment:

- Parallel to a line joining the superior aspect of both acetabulae.

### Coverage:

*Superior to inferior:*
- Superior acetabulum to lesser trochanter

*Lateral to medial:*
- Trochanteric bursae on both sides

*Posterior to anterior:*
- Greater trochanters to anterior acetabulae.

### Demonstrates:

- Bilateral disease processes, such as osteonecrosis.

## Radial
### Position:

- As per routine hip sequences.

### Other considerations:

- Nil.

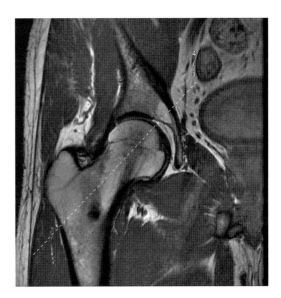

**Figure 6.9** Step 1: Axial oblique planned on a true coronal image.
(North Shore Radiology)

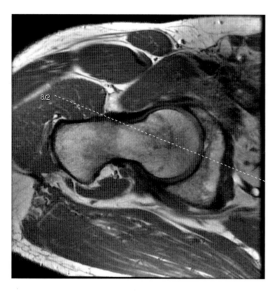

Figure 6.10 Step 2: Planning a coronal double oblique, using the result from Step 1.
(North Shore Radiology)

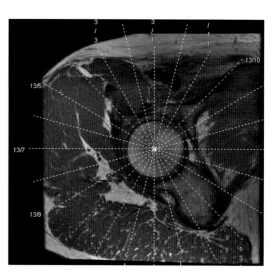

Figure 6.12 Step 4: Planning the radial slices, using the result of Step 3.
(North Shore Radiology)

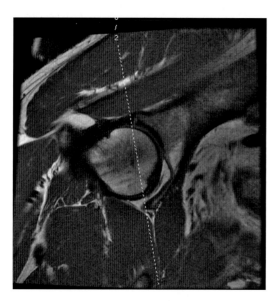

Figure 6.11 Step 3: Planning a third slice, using the result of Step 2.
(North Shore Radiology)

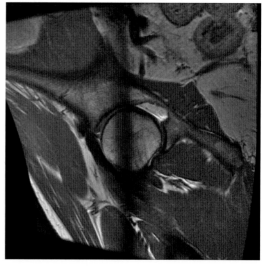

Figure 6.13 A radial image, demonstrating cross excitation from the intersecting slices. Note how the saturated signal passes through the acetabulum, without obscuring the labrum.
(North Shore Radiology)

## Alignment

- Planning requires four steps to ensure the scans radiate around the labrum from its precise centre.
  - Step 1: Using a true coronal image, an axial oblique localiser is planned perpendicular to a line joining both sides of the labral acetabulum (Fig 6.9).
  - Step 2: Using the axial oblique localiser, a second localiser is acquired in a similar manner perpendicular to a line joining both sides of the labral acetabulum, creating a double oblique coronal image (Fig 6.10).
  - Step 3: Using the double oblique coronal image, a final localiser is planned parallel to a line joining the two sides of the labral acetabulum, creating a double oblique coronal image (Fig 6.11).
  - Step 4: The radial images are planned off the final, double oblique coronal image in 15° increments (Fig 6.12).

## Coverage:

*Superior to inferior:*
- Complete coverage of the acetabulum

*Lateral to medial:*
- Acetabulum to mid-femoral neck

*Posterior to anterior:*
- Complete coverage of the articular capsule.

## Coverage:

- Acetabulum to femoral neck.

## Demonstrates:

- Anterosuperior labral tears
- Relationship of bone lesions to the joint
- Due to cross excitation between the slices as they rotate about a central point, each will have a characteristic black line through the centre, as demonstrated in Figure 6.13.

# Chapter 6.2 Quadriceps and hamstring

ONLINE CASE ST
CS2

## Indications:

- Muscle or tendon tear
- Mass.

**A**

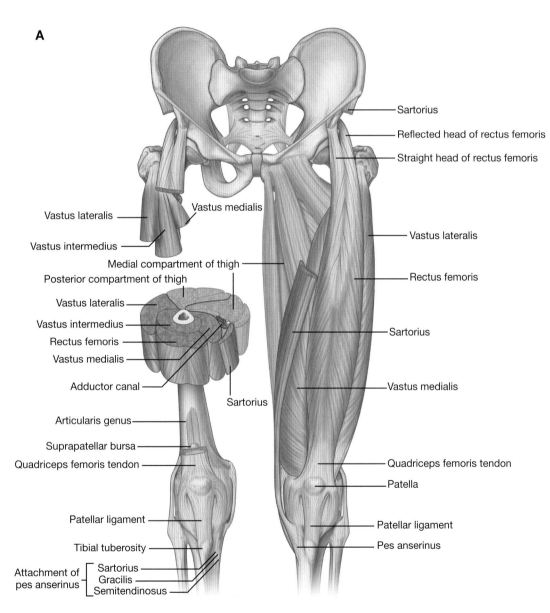

**Figure 6.14** Muscles of the anterior and posterior compartments of the upper leg.
(from Drake, Gray's Anatomy for Students 2e, with permission)

**B**

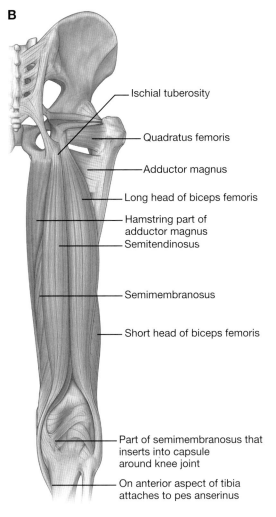

- Ischial tuberosity
- Quadratus femoris
- Adductor magnus
- Long head of biceps femoris
- Hamstring part of adductor magnus
- Semitendinosus
- Semimembranosus
- Short head of biceps femoris
- Part of semimembranosus that inserts into capsule around knee joint
- On anterior aspect of tibia attaches to pes anserinus

Figure 6.14  Continued

## Coils and patient considerations

The quadriceps refer to the four muscles on the anterior aspect of the upper leg, namely the vastus meadialis, intermedius and lateralis, and the rectus femoris; the longest of these is the rectus femoris, originating at the ilium. Deep to this muscle the vastus intermedius originates on the upper antero-medial femur. The vastus medialis arises at the level of the intertrochanteric line from the antero-medial femur, while the vastus lateralis originates near the greater tuberosity. All extend to attach at the patella.

On the posterior aspect of the upper leg, the hamstring is formed by the semimembranosus, semi-tendinosus and biceps femoris muscles. There is close association between their origins at the ischial tuberosity.

Although the quadriceps are on the anterior aspect of the femur and the hamstring is posterior, scanning principles are similar. Being long muscles, imaging with a coil designed for imaging of the pelvis or abdomen permits coverage of the majority of the muscle (Figs I.1 & I.2).

# Imaging planes: Routine sequences

## Position:

- Supine, generally feet first
- Legs flat or at most with a small cushion under the knees to relieve discomfort, resting in a relaxed neutral position
- Hands away from the imaging coils.

## Other considerations:

- When body habitus causes a large coil to slope downwards towards the legs, sponges can level out the coil preventing it from sliding caudally during the examination. This should also assist in producing a consistent signal throughout the images.
- For hamstrings, the musculotendinous junction, extending roughly 12 cm distally, must be included as this is the most common site of injury, particularly for biceps femoris.
- Injuries of the distal hamstring and quadriceps tendon attachments are more appropriately investigated by imaging the knee.

## Coronal

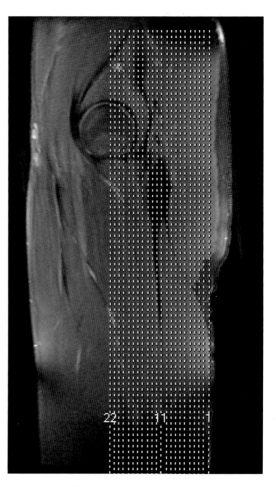

**Figure 6.16** Hamstrings, coronal planned on a sagittal image.
(North Shore Radiology)

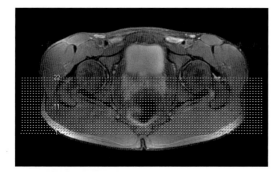

**Figure 6.15** Hamstrings, coronal planned on an axial image.
(North Shore Radiology)

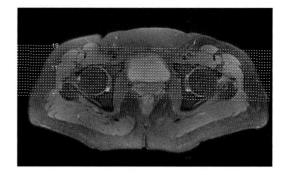

**Figure 6.17** Quadriceps, coronal planned on an axial image.
(North Shore Radiology)

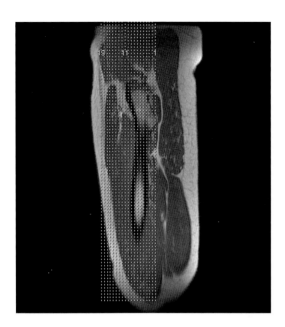

Figure 6.18 Quadriceps, coronal planned on a sagittal image.
(North Shore Radiology)

## Alignment:

- For both the hamstrings and quadriceps, align scans parallel to the femoral heads
- Coronal images will include both legs.

## Coverage:

*Superior to inferior:*
- Hamstrings: ischial tuberosities to mid-femoral shaft
- Quadriceps: anterior superior iliac spine (ASIS) to as far distal as the coil permits

*Lateral to medial:*
- Right to left legs

*Posterior to anterior:*
- Hamstrings: ischial tuberosities and hamstring muscles to mid-femoral shaft
- Quadriceps: mid-femoral shaft and ASIS to anterior quadriceps surface.

## Demonstrates:

- Acquiring long axis images first assists in demonstration of the location and extent of inflammation or disruption of the musculotendinous junctions. Subsequent images can then be targeted to evident pathology.
- If the entire length of the muscle is not imaged in a single field of view and no abnormality is demonstrated, the patient should be repositioned to image the distal portions to ensure no pathology is overlooked.
- Hamstrings:
  - Proximal origin avulsion (rare in adults) and consequential retraction of the conjoint (semitendinosus and biceps femoris) and semimembranous tendons from the ischium.
- Quadriceps:
  - Rectus femoris, vastus lateralis, intermedius and medialis. Differentiation of the individual origins may be better demonstrated in the axial plane.

## Axial

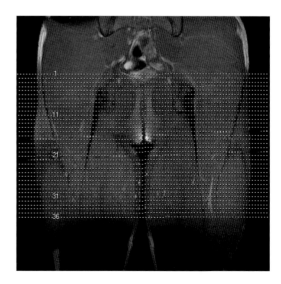

Figure 6.19 Proximal hamstrings, axial planned on a coronal image.
(North Shore Radiology)

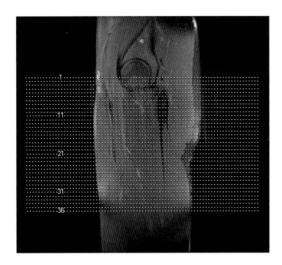

Figure 6.20 Proximal hamstrings, axial planned on a sagittal image.
(North Shore Radiology)

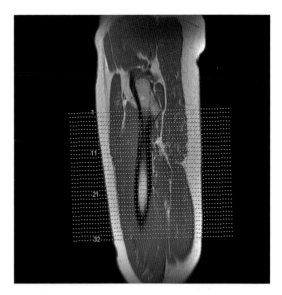

Figure 6.22 Unilateral proximal quadriceps, axial planned on a sagittal image.
(North Shore Radiology)

## Alignment:

- For both the hamstrings and quadriceps, align scans parallel to the femoral heads.

## Coverage:

- As per coronal plane
- For discrete injuries, superoinferior coverage should focus on the pathological region identified on the coronal scans.

## Demonstrates:

- Tendinopathy, indicated by tendon thickening with or without obvious tear or oedema.
- Hamstrings:
  - Origins of the conjoint (biceps femoris and semitendinosis) and semimembranosus tendons and progressive differentiation into the three separate entities.
- Quadriceps:
  - Differentiation of the individual origins of the rectus femoris, vastus lateralis, intermedius and medialis.

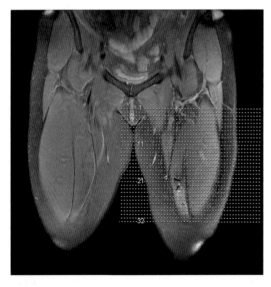

Figure 6.21 Unilateral proximal quadriceps, axial planned on a coronal image.
(North Shore Radiology)

# Imaging planes: Supplementary sequences

## Sagittal

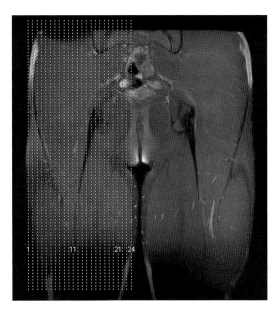

**Figure 6.23** Sagittal hamstrings planned on a coronal image.
(North Shore Radiology)

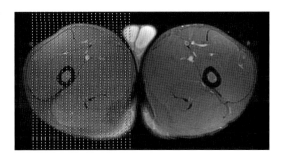

**Figure 6.24** Sagittal upper leg planned on an axial image.
(North Shore Radiology)

## Alignment:

- Planned off a coronal image to include the area of injury.

## Coverage:

*Superior to inferior:*
- Hamstrings: ischial tuberosities to as far distal as signal permits
- Quadriceps: ASIS to as far distal as the coil permits

*Lateral to medial:*
- Lateral to medial skin surfaces

*Posterior to anterior:*
- Posterior to anterior skin surfaces of upper leg.

## Demonstrates:

- Hamstring:
  - Secondary assessment of the hamstring complex
- Quadriceps:
  - Rectus femoris origin at the ASIS
  - Muscle bellies and secondary assessment of the muscles.

# Chapter 6.3 Knee

## Indications:

- Disruption of knee ligaments, i.e. anterior or posterior cruciate ligaments (ACL or PCL), medial or lateral collateral ligaments (MCL or LCL)
- Mensical damage +/– para-meniscal and Baker's cysts
- Patellofemoral disease
- Chondromalacia
- Osteonecrosis (AVN)
- Mass, e.g. giant cell tumour
- Arthritis (OA or RA)
- Synovial disorders, including pigmented villonodualr synovitis (PVNS) or synovial osteochondromatosis (SOC)
- Bursitis of the pes anserinus (also known as goosefoot bursitis).

## Coils and patient considerations

Interposed by the fibrocartilage of the medial and later menisci, the knee joint is stabilised by the anterior and posterior cruciate, collateral, popliteal and transverse ligaments. The sesamoid patella sits within the patella tendon, acting as a fulcrum for the quadriceps muscle, enabling it to bear much greater load than it would otherwise accommodate. All four quadriceps muscles (vastus medialis, inter-medius and lateralis and the rectus femoris) insert at the patella.

Posteriorly, the three muscles of the hamstring diverge with the semitendinosus and semimem-branosus merging with the gracilis to form the pes anserine. This lies superficial to the medial collateral ligament, attaching medial to the tibial tuberosity.

The biceps femoris becomes intimately associated with the lateral collateral ligament and the iliotibial tract, although a single conjoined tendon is not generally formed. It inserts at the fibula head.

Imaging coils are generally cylindrical in nature but the inside may be flat (Fig I.8) or moulded (Fig I.7) to the back of the knee. This needs to be borne in mind, as flexion permits laxity of the ACL and may influence conspicuity of partial tears. In addition, coronal and axial slices will not be truly so in both the proximal and distal joint if the leg is bent. A bend of no more than 10° should be encouraged. In the event that the patient is unable to tolerate extension of the joint, a flexible coil may be used as an alternative (Fig I.11), although this may com-promise both image quality and the demonstration of pathology.

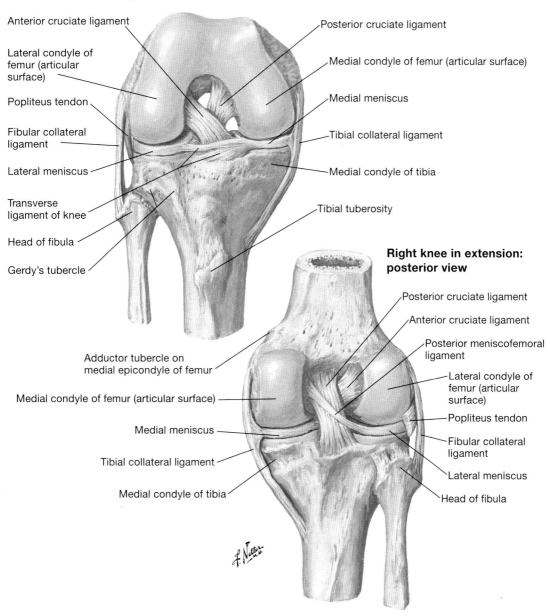

**Right knee in flexion: anterior view**

Anterior cruciate ligament

Lateral condyle of femur (articular surface)

Popliteus tendon

Fibular collateral ligament

Lateral meniscus

Transverse ligament of knee

Head of fibula

Gerdy's tubercle

Posterior cruciate ligament

Medial condyle of femur (articular surface)

Medial meniscus

Tibial collateral ligament

Medial condyle of tibia

Tibial tuberosity

**Right knee in extension: posterior view**

Adductor tubercle on medial epicondyle of femur

Medial condyle of femur (articular surface)

Medial meniscus

Tibial collateral ligament

Medial condyle of tibia

Posterior cruciate ligament

Anterior cruciate ligament

Posterior meniscofemoral ligament

Lateral condyle of femur (articular surface)

Popliteus tendon

Fibular collateral ligament

Lateral meniscus

Head of fibula

**Figure 6.25** The knee joint.
(Netter illustration from www.netterimages.com ©Elsevier Inc. All rights reserved.)

# Imaging planes: Routine sequences

## Position:

- Supine, generally feet first
- Leg straight so that the knee is fully extended or flexed no more than 10° to retain tension on the ACL. Slight flexion reduces meniscal flounce.

## Other considerations:

- Support beneath the knee should be used to ensure no movement
- Inability to fully extend the knee will result in laxity in the ACL, which may affect demonstration of a partial tear.

## Axial

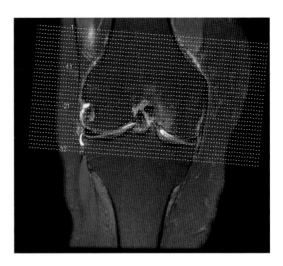

**Figure 6.27** Axial planned on a coronal image. (North Shore Radiology)

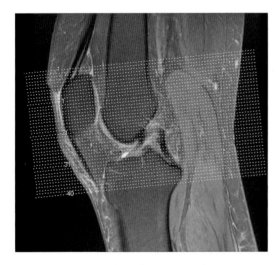

**Figure 6.26** Axial planned on a sagittal image. (North Shore Radiology)

## Alignment:

- Parallel to the inferior aspect of the femoral condyles and the menisci.

## Coverage:

*Superior to inferior:*
- Suprapatellar fat to PCL insertion
- For pes anserinus bursitis, coverage should include the anterior crest of the tibia, where the conjoined tendons of the hamstring attach

*Lateral to medial:*
- Tibiofibular joint to medial joint line

*Posterior to anterior:*
- Posterior to anterior skin surfaces.

## Demonstrates:

- Patella cartilage and trochlear groove
- Medial and lateral collateral ligaments and quadriceps tendon
- Inflammation of the pes anserinus bursa
- Secondary demonstration of circumferential meniscal tears
- Secondary assessment of cruciate ligaments
- Neurovascular structures.

# Coronal

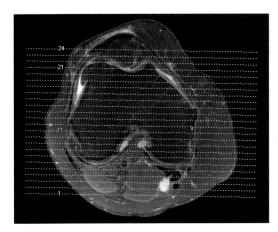

**Figure 6.28** Coronal planned on an axial image. (North Shore Radiology)

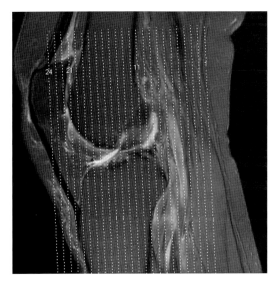

**Figure 6.29** Coronal planned on a sagittal image. (North Shore Radiology)

## Alignment:

- Parallel to a line joining the posterior aspect of the femoral condyles
- If the knee is more than minimally flexed, scans should be perpendicular to the tibial plateau in the sagittal plane to clearly demonstrate the meniscus and ligamentous insertions at the proximal tibia.

## Coverage:

*Superior to inferior:*
- Quadriceps tendon insertion to MCL insertion

*Lateral to medial:*
- Iliotibial tract to MCL

*Posterior to anterior:*
- Popliteal fossa to patella.

## Demonstrates:

- Medial and lateral collateral ligament integrity
- Secondary assessment of cruciate ligament
- Secondary assessment of meniscal pathology
- Femoral and tibial osteochondral integrity.

# Sagittal oblique

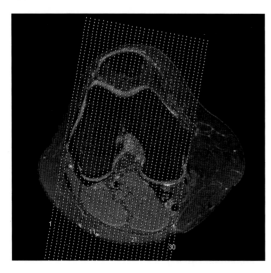

Figure 6.30 Sagittal oblique planned on an axial image.
(North Shore Radiology)

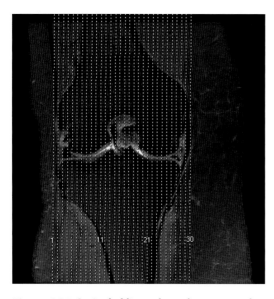

Figure 6.31 Sagittal oblique planned on a coronal image.
(North Shore Radiology)

## Alignment:

· Angled in plane with the ACL on an axial image (requires approximately 10° medial rotation)
· In the case of ruptured ACL, a plane parallel to the lateral aspect of the intercondylar notch on an axial image.

## Coverage:

· As per coronal plane.

## Demonstrates:

· ACL and PCL
· Meniscal pathology, particularly displaced bucket handle tears of the medial meniscus
· Cruciate ligaments
· Pre-patellar bursitis
· Quadriceps and patellar tendon
· Trochlear groove and femoral and tibial osteochondral integrity
· Secondary assessment of patellar cartilage and Hoffa's fat pad
· Secondary demonstration of neurovascular structures.

# Chapter 6.4 Ankle

## Indications:

- Ligamentous or tendinous disruption
- Osteochondral talar dome lesions
- Syndesmosis +/− diastasis injuries
- Osteonecrosis (AVN, Kohler's disease of the navicular)
- Tendinitis, fasciitis, fibromatosis
- Mass, e.g. giant cell tumour, ganglion, lipoma
- Arthritis (OA, RA, inflammatory), gout

- Synovial disorders, including pigmented villonodualr synovitis (PVNS) or synovial osteochondromatosis (SOC)
- Achilles tendon injury +/− Haglund's deformity
- Tarsal coalition
- Impingement syndromes
- Plantar fasciitis and fibromatosis.

## Coils and patient considerations

The ankle is a complex joint stabilised by a range of tendons and ligaments. Comprised of the distal fibula and tibia and the talus, imaging encompasses the calcaneus and the navicular and cuboid. Ligaments can be grouped into three categories. Medially the anterior and posterior tibiotalar, tibionavicular and tibiocalcaneal ligaments, collectively referred to as the deltoid ligament, prevent extreme eversion of the subtalar joint. Supporting the lateral aspect are the anterior and posterior ligaments and calcaneofibular ligaments. The anterior and posterior inferior tibiofibular ligaments, the transverse and the interosseous ligaments form the syndesmosis. These ensure the intimacy of the bones of the lower leg and act to stabilise and transmit load to the fibula.

Overlying the lateral capsule, the tendons of the peroneus brevis and longus course posterior and inferior to the malleolus. Peroneus longus moves medially once it reaches the cuboid, coursing under the metatarsals to attach on the lateral aspect of the first metatarsal and first cuneiform. Peroneus brevis remains lateral and attaches to the base of the fifth metatarsal.

On the medial aspect, the flexor digitorum longus (FDL), flexor hallucis longus (FHL) and posterior tibial tendon (PTT) course behind the malleolus. The FDL divides into four tendons in the sole of the foot, which attach to the bases of the distal phalanges of the second to fifth toes. The FHL slides beneath the sustenaculum tali and extends along the medial sole to insert at the base of the distal phalanx of the great toe. The PTT divides into three tendons, attaching over a broad area to the second to fourth metatarsals bases, the cuneiforms, cuboid, navicular and sustentaculum tali of the calcaneus.

Anteriorly the anterior tibial tendon (ATT) extends over the joint to attach to the medial cuneiform and the first metatarsal, while posteriorly the Achilles tendon extends from the calf to attach to the calcaneus.

Imaging coils for examining the ankle are moulded to the joint (Figs I.8 & I.9). The sharp change in angle of the tendons as they pass from the lower leg into the joint makes them subject to the effects of magic angle. Positioning the foot in a relaxed position (up to 20° flexion) minimises the effects of magic angle. Hyperflexion of the joint also narrows the anterior joint capsule and is undesirable.

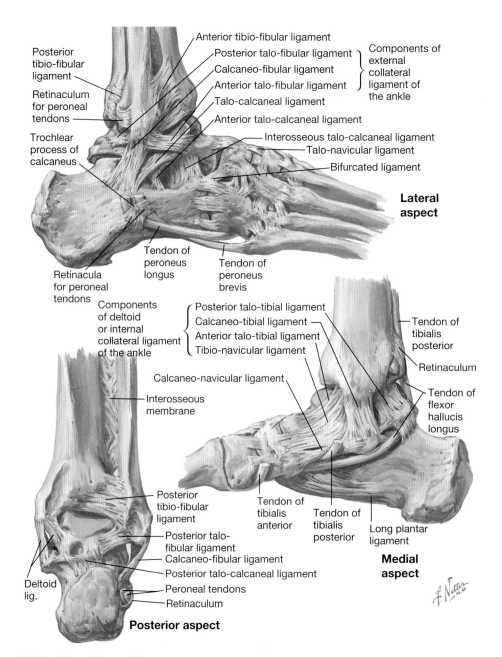

Figure 6.32 Ankle tendons and ligaments.

(Netter illustration from www.netterimages.com ©Elsevier Inc. All rights reserved.)

# Imaging planes: Routine sequences

## Position:

- Supine, generally feet first
- Leg straight, supported at the knee
- Foot flexed up to 20°
- A small sponge under the knee may alleviate lower back pain.

## Other considerations:

- Extreme plantar flexion is discouraged.

## Sagittal

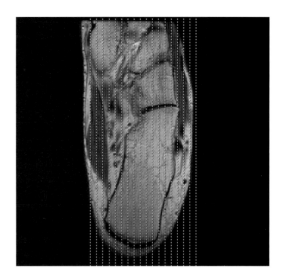

Figure 6.34 Sagittal planned on an axial image. (North Shore Radiology)

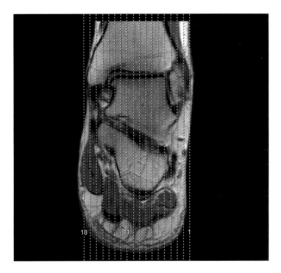

Figure 6.33 Sagittal planned on a coronal image. (North Shore Radiology)

## Alignment:

- Perpendicular to the talar dome in the coronal plane
- Parallel to the long axis of the lower leg.

## Coverage:

*Superior to inferior:*
- Distal quarter of tibia to sole of foot
- For Achilles tendon, include the musculotendinous junction (at least 8 cm above insertion)

*Lateral to medial:*
- Fibula to medial malleolus

*Posterior to anterior:*
- Posterior skin edge to base of fifth metatarsal.

## Demonstrates:

- Subtalar joints best demonstrated in this plane
- Achilles tendon
- Talar dome, sinus tarsi and tarsal morphology
- Disruption of the anterior and posterior ligaments and tendons
- Proximal peroneus brevis and longus tendons posteroinferior to the lateral malleolus. These may be tracked to their insertions at the base of the fifth and inferolateral aspect of the first metatarsal base, respectively.
- FHL, FDL and PTT can be tracked on the medial aspect, although the insertion points are beyond the tarsals (see Ch 6.5).
- Os trigonum
- Plantar fascia (aponeurosis) +/− calcaneal spurs
- Neural structures within the tarsal tunnel.

# Axial

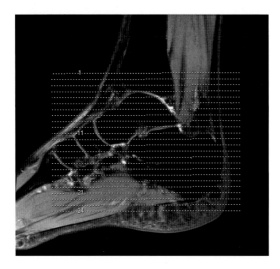

Figure 6.35 Axial planned on a sagittal image.
(North Shore Radiology)

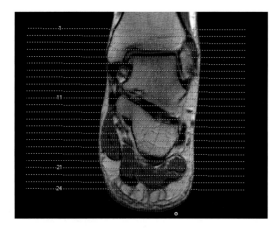

Figure 6.36 Axial planned on a coronal image.
(North Shore Radiology)

## Alignment:

· Parallel to the talar dome and the plantar fascia.

## Coverage:

*Superior to inferior:*
· Epiphyseal plate of the distal tibia to the plantar fascia
· For Achilles tendon, include the musculotendinous junction. This may require separate imaging of the distal calf above the ankle joint to ensure sufficient signal, especially if the tendon is torn and retracted.

*Lateral to medial:*
· Fibula to medial malleolus

*Posterior to anterior:*
· Achilles insertion to the base of fifth metatarsal.

## Demonstrates:

· Tendon morphology and injury
· Sinus tarsi and neurovascular structures
· Syndesmosis injuries
· Dislocation of medial and lateral tendons and ligaments
· Achilles tendon and FHL
· Fracture/avulsion of the peroneus brevis from the base of the fifth metatarsal and tarsal stress injuries
· Tarsal coalition
· Spring ligament complex.

# Coronal

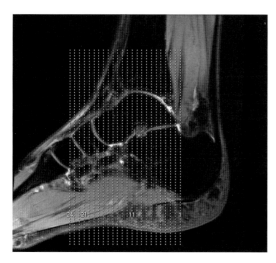

Figure 6.37 Coronal planned on a sagittal image. (North Shore Radiology)

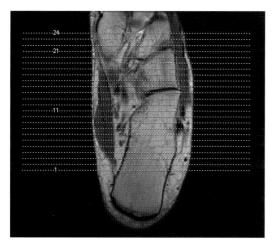

Figure 6.38 Coronal planned on an axial image. (North Shore Radiology)

## Alignment:

- Perpendicular to the long axis of the distal tibia.

## Coverage:

*Superior to inferior:*
- Distal quarter of tibia to dorsum of foot
- For Achilles tendon, include the musculotendinous junction (at least 8 cm above insertion)

*Lateral to medial:*
- Fibula to medial malleolus

*Posterior to anterior:*
- Posterior articular facet of calcaneus to the cuneiforms
- For Achilles tendon, posterior skin edge to talonavicular junction.

## Coverage:

- As for axial plane.

## Demonstrates:

- Best plane for examining tibiotalar joint
- Plantar fascia (aponeurosis)
- Malleoli and talus
- Distal medial and lateral ankle ligaments
- Subtalar joint, especially for talocalcaneal coalition
- Sinus tarsi and tarsal tunnel disruption
- Anterolateral impingement
- Spring ligament complex.

# Chapter 6.5 Midfoot

## Indications:

- Lisfranc injury (disruption of the articulation between the second and third metatarsal bases, with or without fracture)
- Midfoot pain
- Mass, e.g. synovial sarcoma is a common malignancy in this area
- Arthopathies, including Charcot foot (neuropathic arthropathy), and the

osteogenic arthropathies, such as gout and RA
- Osteonecrosis (AVN)
- Osteomyelitis.
- Osteoarthritis (OA)
- Tarsal stress injury.

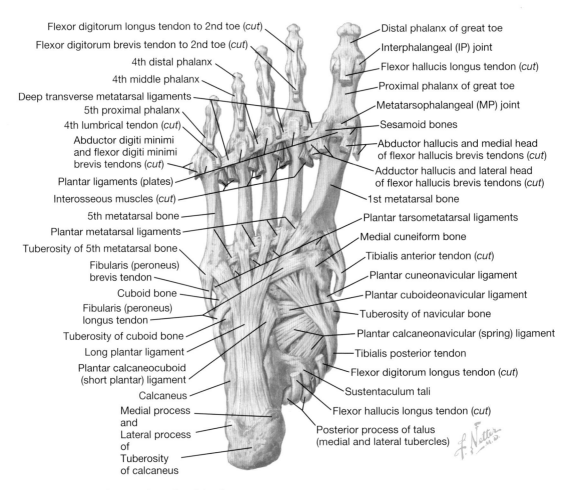

**Figure 6.39** Tendons in the sole of the foot.
(Netter illustration from www.netterimages.com ©Elsevier Inc. All rights reserved.)

# Coils and patient considerations

Imaging of the midfoot encompasses the bones of the navicular, cuboid, proximal metatarsals and the cuneiforms. The cuneiforms articulate with the bases of the first to third metatarsals, with the Lisfranc ligament extending from the medial cuneiform anterolaterally to the posteromedial aspect of the base of the second metatarsal. This stabilises the joint between the first and second metatarsals. The cuboid articulates with the bases of the fourth and fifth metatarsals. Many of the tendons mentioned in Chapter 6.4 on the ankle attach to the bases of the metatarsals of the cuneiforms.

Use of an imaging coil similar to those shown in Chapter 6.4 is possible, but an altered position may be required. Imaging with the foot plantar is preferred to ameliorate potential issues with magic angle artefacts. Positioning with the knee bent over a bolster and the foot in plantar flexion may be preferred. The heel must be supported so that the foot does not slip out of the coil posteriorly. Alternately, the patient may be imaged prone with the ventral aspect of the foot resting in the coil. Whichever position is adopted, pack the coil with MRI safe sponges to assist with immobilisation.

Confusion over plane designations is common when imaging beyond the talocalcaneal joint. Assuming the foot is dorsiflexed, anatomical position places the long axis of the metatarsals in the axial (transverse) plane. This concept is counter-intuitive compared to the rest of the body for which the length of a long bone is generally demonstrated in the coronal plane. To alleviate confusion, the terms short and long axis (described relative to the metatarsals) will be employed in this chapter to describe slice orientations. The term sagittal refers to imaging in a parasagittal or sagittal oblique plane.

Slice orientations used for the ankle are inappropriate beyond the talocalcanleal joint. The curvature induced by the longitudinal arch means that compound obliquity is necessary to effectively demonstrate joints between the navicular and metatarsals. Prescribing scans in the order listed in this chapter, each from the previous dataset, will enable creation of the necessary double oblique images.

# Imaging planes: Routine sequences

## Position:

- Supine, generally feet first
- Knees bent, supported by a bolster
- Foot plantar in the imaging coil.

## Other considerations:

- If the patient is unable to maintain the desired degree of flexion, compromise will need to be made. Use sponges to support the sole of the foot and immobilise on the ventral and lateral aspects.
- Some patients may prefer to be imaged prone.

## Short axis

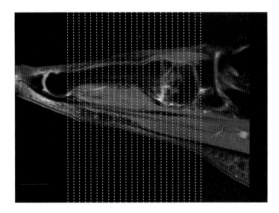

Figure 6.40 Short axis planned on a sagittal image.
(North Shore Radiology)

## Alignment:

- Perpendicular to the shaft of the metatarsals in the sagittal and coronal planes.

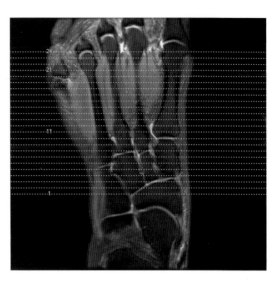

Figure 6.41 Short axis planned on a long axis image.
(North Shore Radiology)

## Coverage:

*Superior to inferior:*
- Navicular-cuneiform joint to heads of the metatarsals
- When pathology is known to be localised to the tarsals, coverage from the talonavicular joint to the midshaft of the metatarsals may be more appropriate.

*Lateral to medial:*
- First to fifth metatarsals

*Posterior to anterior:*
- Dorsum to ventral aspect of the foot.

## Demonstrates:

- Tissue contour and signal changes around and within each metatarsal
- Tarsometatarsal disruption.

# Long axis

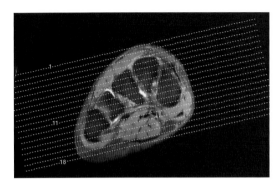

Figure 6.42 Long axis planned on a short axis image.
(North Shore Radiology)

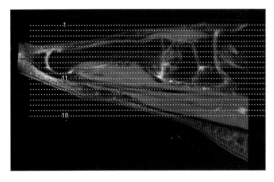

Figure 6.43 Long axis planned on a sagittal image.
(North Shore Radiology)

## Alignment:

- Planned from the completed short axis series so as to achieve the compound double obliquity
- For imaging of the tarsals and tarsometatarsal joints:
  - Parallel to a line joining the base of the first to fourth metatarsals
- For imaging of the metatarsals:
  - Parallel to the line joining the midshafts of the first to fourth metatarsals.

## Coverage:

- As for short axis
- If pathology is localised to the tarsals, distal coverage to the midshaft of the metatarsals may be sufficient.

## Demonstrates:

- Tarso-metatarsal disruption
- Malalignment of the joints of the proximal foot.

# Sagittal

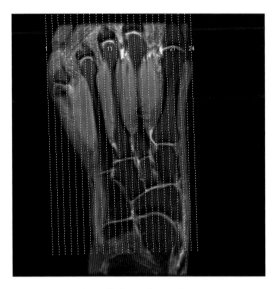

Figure 6.44 Sagittal planned on a long axis image. (North Shore Radiology)

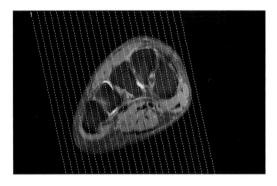

Figure 6.45 Sagittal planned on a short axis image. (North Shore Radiology)

## Alignment:

- Planned from the completed short and long axis series so as to achieve the compound double obliquity
- For imaging of the tarsal and tarsometatarsal joints:
  - Perpendicular to a line joining the base of the first to fourth metatarsals
- For imaging of the metatarsals:
  - Perpendicular to the line joining the midshafts of the first to fourth metatarsals and along the long bone of interest.

## Coverage:

- As for the short axis
- If pathology is localised to the tarsals, distal coverage to the midshaft of the metatarsals may be sufficient.

## Demonstrates:

- Tarsometatarsal disruption
- Collapse of the plantar arch.

# Chapter 6.6 Forefoot and toes

## Indications:

- Mass, e.g Morton's neuroma, giant cell tumour of the tendon sheath (PVNS), granulomas, ganglions
- Turf toe or ligamentous disruption of the first metatarsophalangeal joint
- Sesamoid injury at the first metatarsophalangeal joint
- Osteomyelitis
- Osteonecrosis of metatarsal heads, e.g. Freiburg's infraction or AVN, most frequently second and third metatarsals
- Stress fractures of the metatarsal neck (March fracture)
- Arthritis (OA and RA).

## Coils and patient considerations

Imaging of the forefoot encompasses the distal metatarsals and the phalanges. Positioning the patient prone has been shown to improve the conspicuity and location of neuromas greater than 5 mm in diameter. Movement artefact is diminished and the toes are plantar flexed, aligning them with the long axis of the metatarsals. A coil designed for extremity work may be used (Figs I.7 & I.8). Small paired dual coils may also be an option when focusing on a particular joint (Fig I.12).

As the arch of the midfoot reduces distally and the curvature continues medially, orientation of the slices needs to be focused on the forefoot, not the midfoot or ankle. Prescribing scans in the order listed in this chapter, each from the previous dataset, will enable creation of the necessary double oblique images. Similar to the terminology used for the midfoot, slice orientation in this chapter is described in terms of short axis, long axis and sagittal.

# Imaging planes: Routine sequences

## Position:

- Prone, generally feet first
- Leg straight
- Ventral surface of forefoot resting within the imaging coil.

## Other considerations:

- If the patient is unable to maintain the desired degree of flexion, the supine position may be used, positioning in a similar manner to the midfoot. Ensure that the metatarsophalangeal joints and phalanges are within the sensitive area of the coil.

## Short axis

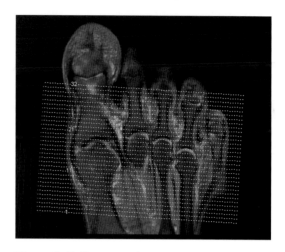

**Figure 6.47** Short axis planned on a long axis image.
(North Shore Radiology)

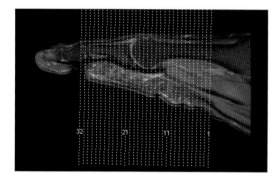

**Figure 6.46** Short axis planned on a sagittal image.
(North Shore Radiology)

## Alignment:

- Transverse to the long axis of the metatarsophalangeal joint.

## Coverage:

*Superior to inferior:*
- For suspected Morton's neuroma and sesamoid injuries, from the metatarsophalangeal joints to the first interphalangeal joints
- For other injuries and degenerative conditions, scans should continue distally to include the whole of the digit(s) of interest

*Lateral to medial:*
- First to fifth metatarsals

*Posterior to anterior:*
- Dorsum to ventral aspect of the foot.

## Demonstrates:

- Intermetatarsal spaces
- Tissue contour and signal changes around and within each metatarsal.

# Long axis

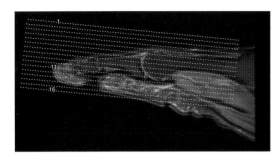

**Figure 6.48** Long axis planned on a sagittal image.
(North Shore Radiology)

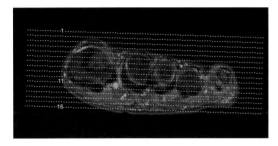

**Figure 6.49** Long axis planned on a short axis image.
(North Shore Radiology)

## Alignment:

- Parallel to a line joining the first to fourth metatarsal heads and the long axis of the first phalanx of the digit(s) of interest
- For great toe sesamoids scans should be aligned to the metatarsal.

## Coverage:

- As for short axis
- Scans should include the tips of the toes.

## Demonstrates:

- Intermetatarsal spaces
- Cortical integrity of the metatarsophalangeal joints.

# Sagittal

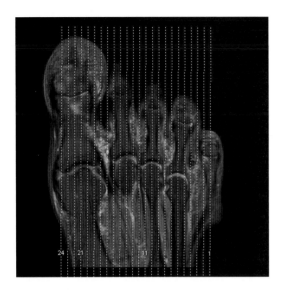

Figure 6.50 Sagittal planned on a long axis image. (North Shore Radiology)

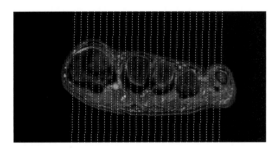

Figure 6.51 Sagittal planned on a short axis image. (North Shore Radiology)

## Alignment:

- To the joint or long bone of interest.

## Coverage:

- As for short axis
- Scans should include the tips of the toes.

## Demonstrates:

- Sesamoid integrity
- Cortical integrity of the metatarsophalangeal joints.

# Further reading

Ali M, Chen TS, Crues JV 2006 MRI of the foot. Applied Radiology 35(12):10–20

Beltran J 1994 Sinus tarsi syndrome. MRI Clinics of North America 2(1):59–65

Bencardino JT, Rosenberg ZS, Brown RR et al 2000 Traumatic musculotendinous injuries of the knee: Diagnosis with MR imaging. Radiographics 20:S103–S120

Benjamin M, Toumi H, Ralphs JR et al 2006 Where tendons and ligaments meet bone: Attachment sites ('entheses') in relation to exercise and/or mechanical load. Journal of Anatomy 208:471–490

Chandnani VP, Bradley YC 1994 Achilles tendon and miscellaneous tendon lesions. MRI Clinics of North America 2(1):89–96

Comacho MA 2004 The double line posterior cruciate ligament sign. Radiology 233:503–504

Cvitanic O, Henzie G, Skezas N et al 2004 MRI diagnosis of tears of the hip abductor tendons (gluteus medius and gluteus minimus). American Journal of Roentgenology 182:137–143

De Smet AA, Best TM 2000 MR imaging of the distribution and location of acute hamstring injuries in athletes. American Journal of Roentgenology 174:393–399

Duke Othopaedics 2009 Wheeless' Textbook of Anatomy. Online. Available: http://www. wheelessonline.com/, 14 Mar 2011

El-Khoury GY, Brandser EA, Saltzman CL 1994 MRI of tendon injuries. Iowa Orthopaedic Journal 14:65–80

Filigenzi JM, Bredella MA 2008 MR imaging of femoroacetabular impingement. Applied Radiology 37(4). Online. Available: http:// www.medscape.com/viewarticle/573242, 14 Mar 2011

Finkel JE 1994 Tarsal tunnel syndrome. MRI Clinics of North America 2(1):67–78

Gabriel H, Fitzgerald SW, Myers MT et al 1994 MR imaging of hip disorders. Radiographics 14:763–781

Hermans JJ, Beumer A, de Jong TAW et al 2010 Anatomy of the distal syndesmosis in adults: A pictorial essay with a multimodality approach. Journal of Anatomy (217):633–645

Herring C 1997 Nomenclature for imaging of the feet. American Journal of Roentgenology 168:277–278

Ho CP, Marks PH, Steadman JR 1999 MR imaging of knee anterior cruciate ligament and associated injuries in skiers. MRI Clinics of North America 7(1):117–130

Hong RJ, Hughes TH, Gentili A et al 2008 Magnetic resonance imaging of the hip. Journal of Magnetic Resonance Imaging 27(3):435–445

Horii M, Kubo T, Hirasawa, Y 2000 Radial MRI of the hip with moderate osteoarthritis. Journal of Bone and Joint Surgery 82-B(3):364–368

James SLJ, Ali K, Malara F et al 2006 MRI findings of femoroacetabular impingement. American Journal of Roentgenology 187:1412–1419

Koulouris G, Connell D 2005 Hamstring muscle complex: An imaging review. Radiographics 25:571–586

Mengiardi B, Zanetti M, Schottle PB et al 2005 Spring ligament complex: MR imaging–anatomic correlation and findings in asymptomatic subjects. Radiology 237:242–249

Norkus SA, Floyd RT 2001 The anatomy and mechanisms of syndesmotic ankle sprains. Journal of Athletic Training 36(1):68–73

Park JS, Ryu KN, Yoon KH 2006 Meniscal flounce on knee MRI: Correlation with meniscal locations after positional changes. American Journal of Roentgenology 187: 364–370

Resnick D, Kang HS 1996 Magnetic resonance imaging: typical protocols. In: Internal derangements of joints. WB Saunders, Philadelphia, pp 35–45

Rubin DA, Towers JD, Britton CA 1995 MR imaging of the foot: Utility of complex oblique imaging planes. American Journal of Roentgenology 166(5):1079–1084

Silder A, Heiderscehit B, Thelen DG et al 2008 MR observation of long-term musculotendon remodeling following a hamstring strain injury. Skeletal Radiology 37(12)1101–1109

Stoller DW 2007 Magnetic resonance imaging in orthopaedics and sports medicine, 3rd edn. Lippincott, Williams & Wilkins, Baltimore, pp 42–97, 307–362, 734–804

Sundberg TP, Toomayan GA, Major NM 2006 Evaluation of the acetabular labrum at 3.0-T MR imaging compared with 1.5-T MR arthrography. Radiology 238(2):706–711

University of Michigan Medical School 2000 Anatomy Tables—Joints of the Upper and Lower Limbs. Online. Available: http://anatomy.med. umich.edu/musculoskeletal_system/joints_ tables.html, 14 Mar 2011

Vande Berg BC, Malghem J, Poilvache P et al 2005 Meniscal tears with fragments displaced in the notch and recesses of knee: MR imaging with arthroscopic comparison. Radiology 234:842–850

Weishaupt D, Treiber K, Kundert H et al 2003 Morton neuroma: MR imaging in prone, supine, and upright weight-bearing body positions. Radiology 226:849–856

Weiss LK, Morehouse HT, Levy IM 1991 Sagittal MR images of the knee: A low-signal band parallel to the posterior cruciate ligament caused by a displaced bucket-handle tear. American Journal of Roentgenology 156:117–119

Zanetti M, Weishaupt D 2005 MR imaging of the forefoot: Morton neuroma and differential diagnoses. Seminars in Musculoskeletal Radiology 9(3):175–186

Zehava SR, Beltran J, Bencardino JT 2000 MR imaging of the ankle and foot. Radiographics 20:S153–S179

# Index

Page numbers followed by 'f' indicates figures, and 't' indicates tables.